The Dictionary of
MODERN HERBALISM

A Comprehensive Guide to Practical Herbal Therapy

Compiled and written by
SIMON MILLS

MJF BOOKS
NEW YORK

Note to the reader: This book is intended as an informational guide. The remedies, approaches, and techniques described herein are meant to supplement, and not to be a substitute for, professional medical care or treatment. They should not be used to treat a serious ailment without prior consultation with a qualified health care professional.

Published by MJF Books
Fine Communications
Two Lincoln Square
60 West 66th Street
New York, NY 10023

ISBN 1-56731-223-3
The Dictionary of Modern Herbalism
Copyright © 1988 Simon Mills

This edition published by arrangement with Healing Arts Press.

Manufactured in the United States of America on acid-free paper

MJF Books and the MJF colophon are trademarks of Fine Creative Media, Inc.

10 9 8 7 6 5 4 3 2 1

DEDICATION
For Margaret, Daniel and Bridget.

INTRODUCTION

These are indeed interesting times. In a world that has for long dedicated itself to the pursuit of technological advancement and scientific precision, it is astonishing to realize that the most ancient form of medicine of all is coming back: herbal medicine is in the throes of a renaissance.

A form of treatment so ancient that its misty origins pre-date humanity is returning to challenge the assumptions of the most sophisticated system of medicine in the world's history, just when that system appears to be at its most dazzling, inventive and powerful. It is easy enough to explain the preponderance of traditional medicine in the underdeveloped world, where as the World Health Organization has admitted, only 15 per cent of the population has access to modern western-style health care services; it is easy enough to explain the continued reliance on plant-derived drugs in countries of the communist bloc unwilling to engage in the capitalist machinations of the western pharmaceutical industry. But how does one explain the persistent and increasing use of plant medicines among most peoples of continental Europe, the welter of books and articles on herbs and the rapidly-increasing retail sales of herbal remedies in the English-speaking western world, as well as the new interest being shown by pharmacists and doctors in herbal remedies and phytotherapy everywhere?

It must surely be that plant remedies are filling a need left unprovided for in modern health care: they are safer, more accessible, and most of all they allow everyone to take charge once more of their own health care. Certainly there seems to be a great thirst for information (once transmitted within families and communities) that may allow us to rediscover traditional healing techniques, imbued as these are with immemorial values of health and wholeness. It is even more exciting when modern research shows that these time-worn techniques are often very effective approaches to the illnesses of the present day.

Yet, in response to a heartfelt need, the real information on herbs has

7

been slow in coming. While it is clear that plants are now seen as accessible and safer alternatives to synthetic drugs, it is less well-known that, in skilled hands, they can provide a coherent and effective alternative to professional medical practice as well, that with the appropriate approaches it is possible to transform them into very powerful curative agents indeed.

The problem has been that the skilled techniques of herbal practitioners throughout the ages were acquired by apprenticeship and practical experience, mostly in rural areas far removed from the academic world of western urbanization. It is only in a few parts of the world that professional medical herbalists have survived the move to the urban environment (the National Institute of Medical Herbalists in the United Kingdom arose in 1864 out of such a move during the Industrial Revolution). These practitioners operate a system that is radically different from modern western medicine (although the best modern features are now incorporated in their diagnoses and interpretations). It can provide coherent approaches to even the most serious diseases, even those which appear to be largely modern in character. It is exciting, vital, positively health-enhancing and, above all, effective.

This book is an attempt to briefly capture some of that traditional approach. It is based on the practical experience and wisdom of medical herbalists working in the Anglo-American tradition. It describes the use of herbs as understood by those who have spent their working lives proving them in practice. All this is tied in with modern research into herbal medicine, to pick out that which really stands the test of time.

How to Use this Book
Compared with the conventional approach, herbal medicine has quite a different emphasis. It uses remedies that are different in their action on the body: in most cases they are geared to supporting the powerful vital recuperative and defensive forces of the body against pathogenic influences, rather than attacking the disease directly.

The entries in this book have been carefully framed with this orientation in mind. One's approach to them will vary with the type of enquiry made:

1. *Herbs* are described in terms of their functional effects on the body wherever possible, rather than in terms of symptoms; the applications provided are only those for which the herbs are most often used, rather than specific or limiting instructions; this is simply because herbs work best if their positive character is appreciated first. To understand how they are best applied, it may be necessary to refer to:

2. *Symptoms and diseases:* these are briefly described and the herbalist's approach to them sketched in; possible remedies are provided for each approach, but often therapeutic classifications are mentioned instead. Both are cross-referenced **in bold type**.

3. *Therapeutic classifications* of remedies (e.g. astringent, bitter, diuretic, laxative, anti-inflammatory or circulatory stimulant) are a key feature in this text. Each classification is defined so as to allow an insight into the specifically herbal approach to treatment, and examples of herbs in each classification are listed.

4. *Other* miscellaneous entries are listed to provide supporting information.

The reader is thus strongly encouraged to follow up the extensive system of cross-referencing to elicit the required information.

Dosages and Preparation
The preparation of herbs for medicinal use is often a skilled practice, requiring a considerable degree of practical training. For home use the infusion and decoction are described and other techniques are briefly defined. However, for each herb a general dosage is all that is provided, typically '1-4 grams of dried herb equivalent three times per day'. The word 'equivalent' means that whatever the preparation used it should contain the equivalent of that amount of herb.

A Final Note

This book is designed as an interpretation of herbal medicine based on the practical experience of expert medical herbalists. *It is not an instruction manual.* No responsibility can be accepted by the author or publishers for the application of any of the enclosed information in practice. In any but the simplest or shortest-term problem advice should be sought from qualified herbal practitioners if herbs are to be considered.

This is an English language guide to herbalism. It mentions certain laws pertaining to the purchase of herbs and the practice of herbal medicine in the United Kingdom. As these same laws do not apply in the United States, the American reader is advised to consult local sources for current regulations governing the use of herbal products. Inquiries may be directed to the individuals and organizations listed at the back of this book under 'Useful Addresses'.

A

---

abortifacient, a drug that induces an abortion, euphemistically referred to in earlier times as an **emmenogogue**. It is illegal for anyone except a registered doctor to knowingly prescribe any agent to a pregnant woman that may terminate her pregnancy. Apart from legal, ethical or moral concerns, there is the practical one that many emmenogogue herbs damage the foetus rather than completely terminating the pregnancy. Plants that may harm during pregnancy include rue, arbor-vitae, sage, juniper, barberry, cinchona, black cohosh, blue cohosh, greater celandine, poke root, blood root, meadow saffron, wormwood and other members of the Artemisia genus, male fern, cotton-root bark, tansy, American mandrake, pennyroyal, therapeutic doses of marjoram, oregano, thyme and rosemary and all **anthraquinone laxatives**. In general it is unwise to treat a pregnant woman with *any* herb unless it has been positively cleared as safe: if at all possible, a professional medical herbalist should be consulted to make the final choice.

---

abortion, threatened *see* **miscarriage.**

---

abscess is a localized collection of pus. On the skin: pustule, **boil,** or carbuncle; on the finger: whitlow; on the jaw: gumboil. Can also develop internally in the breast, kidney, brain and abdomen. All but the most simple should be referred for treatment and possible drainage, and some may be positively dangerous if neglected. There is a generalized form known as erysipelas. Chronic abscesses are often tubercular and should not be treated casually either.

Acacia catechu, catechu, black.

Achillea millefolium, yarrow.

---

acne, overactivity of the sebaceous glands of the skin. Usually reflecting fluctuations in sex hormone levels and activity, as in adolescent development. Dietary measures should emphasize the elimination of chocolate, beef and pork products, fats, sweets, nuts and spices and the consumption of lots of fresh fruit, raw vegetables and fluids. Tea and coffee should also be controlled. Treatment will concentrate on using **eliminative** remedies, checking that bowel function in particular is adequate. Where the condition persists after adolescence then hormonal **adaptogens** may have to be considered.

---

acne rosacea, or rosacea, is a condition of dilation of blood vessels to the face leading to a congested flushing affecting the cheeks and nose; can be intermittent and mild, or chronic and with severe damage to the skin. Most often associated with disturbed digestion (*see* **dyspepsia**) and hormonal upset, especially during menopause. Alcohol and tea are exacerbatory. The herbalist emphasizes remedies for digestion and liver function as appropriate, and will seek to balance hormonal disturbances if needed, *see* **hormonal remedies.**

---

aconite, Monkshood, Wolfsbane, *Aconitum napelus* L. Fam: Ranunculaceae

The root of a perennial herb with striking dark-blue, helmet-shaped flowers arranged in a spike up to 150cm tall; the root is tuberous with, each year, a new tuber displacing its predecessors; the leaves are characteristically divided.

Habitat: native to central and southern Europe in moist rich meadows; cultivated as an ornamental elsewhere.

Constituents: alkaloids (including aconitine, aconine, ephedrine and sparteine).

Action: the alkaloids act to drastically reduce nerve activity, but also to stimulate the heart and circulation; it is one of the most toxic plants available but has been used traditionally in minute doses as an anodyne and circulatory stimulant.

Applications: to neuralgia, sciatica and other nerve pains and rheumatic pain as a topical application; for the local treatment of bruises and contusions.

Dosage: the lotion must not contain more than 1.3 parts of aconite to 100 parts of lotion, under restrictions imposed in the 1968 Medicines Act.

Caution: the effective dose is so close to the toxic level that this remedy is not to be used internally; even external application must be over unbroken skin and careful observation made as to toxic side-effects from excessive absorption.

Aconitum napelus,   aconite.

Acorus calamus,   sweet flag.

---

acrid constituents,   a term used to describe those plant constituents that are 'hot' to taste: thus components of the hot spices. They are a heterogenous group in chemical terms but all have the ability to produce transient inflammation on exposed mucous surfaces: the 'hot' sensation is produced by pain fibres involved in that reaction. The histamine-like effect is usually transferred to the interior when the substances are absorbed, accounting for a rise in body temperature and a subjective sensation of warmth. It is established that there is also a general increase in blood flow through the tissues. The acrid effect has been used by herbalists as a central tool in their strategy of repelling disease, especially those traditionally linked with 'cold', like respiratory and some enteric infections and fevers. In modern times the acrid principle is widely used by practitioners wherever sluggish or congested circulation is suspected as the root of a problem. Notable examples of plants used for this effect include cayenne, ginger, horseradish, raw garlic, and mustard. *See* **circulatory stimulants.**

---

active principle,   that constituent of a herb or other medicine which is judged on pharmacological evidence to be the most active. It is then typically isolated and possibly synthesized to provide the basis for a standardized drug, notable examples including aspirin, digoxin, ephedrine, morphine and codeine. These isolates are thought to be more predictable than when found as part of a complex package. The herbalist disagrees fundamentally with this approach. The herbal pharmacologist points to the evidence of interaction that occurs between constituents in the whole plant to produce effects not found when any single one is taken in isolation;

to the evidence that people vary widely in their reaction to even the most standardized drug, and to the central point that herbs are applied for different reasons to drugs anyway (*see* **herbalism**). It is the herbal contention that, in those select plants tried and proven by use through the ages, the balance of constituents in the whole cannot be mimicked by isolating any individual fragments, that the whole is truly more than the sum of its parts.

---

adaptogen, literally means a remedy that improves adaptability. This is a term that has been applied to remedies that appear to help maintain an adequate 'stress response' as defined by the physiologist Hans Selye. Many have followed him in seeing a root cause for many chronic degenerative diseases in a reduced ability of the body to 'rise to' the many stresses we are all exposed to through life, this being seen in turn as an exhaustion of the adrenal cortex stress hormone response leading to a loss of adaptability in body function. Interest has thus been generated by the observation that some remedies actually seem to help maintain and improve adrenal stress response: they include the Asiatic and Siberian ginsengs and other less well investigated members of that family, and dong quai and gotu kola. The term 'adaptogen' is also increasingly used to denote a common quality of herbal remedies, that is their ability to help a function or system so as to improve apparently contradictory symptoms: such remedies can be seen as centrally supportive in their action. Examples are helonias root and agnus-castus for the female hormonal system, blue cohosh and life root for the uterus, hawthorn for the heart, the **bitters** for the pancreatic hormones and liver function, garlic and limeflowers for the peripheral circulation, garlic also for the gut flora, linseed and the **aperients** for the bowel, yarrow for the fever mechanism, ground ivy for upper respiratory mucous membrane function, and oats for the central nervous system. An examination of many other remedies will provide indications that such restorative activity is surprisingly common.

Addison's disease, a condition of atrophy of the cells in the adrenal cortex producing the stress hormones (such as cortisone) and other steroids. The symptoms are severe anaemia and debility, wasting and pigmentation of the skin. Although initially described in 1855 it has become more common as a result of over-prescription of steroid drugs. A case has been reported of the condition being reversed with the administration of large amounts of licorice.

---

adenoids, protective lymphatic glands at the back of the nasal cavity and throat. Mainly noticed when enlarged, especially in children when they obstruct breathing through the nose. Removal should be considered a measure of last resort however: there are adequate herbal approaches available for most cases, *see* **tonsillitis** and **catarrh.**

Aesculus hippocastanum, chestnut, horse.

Agathosma betulina, buchu.

agnus-castus, Chasteberry, Monk's Pepper, *Vitex agnus-castus* L., Fam: Verbenaceae.

The fruit of a densely branched shrub up to 5cm in height; the fruit appears after whorls of violet flowers on long terminal shoots.

Habitat: indigenous to the Mediterranean countries and Asia.

Constituents: a volatile oil, alkaloids, and a bitter principle, castine.

Action: the volatile oil acts on the anterior pituitary, tending to increase the production of luteotrophic hormone leading to a restoration of corpus luteum function; there is an increase in milk production during lactation.

Applications: to menstrual problems resulting from corpus luteum deficiency, particularly those marked by premenstrual symptoms, spasmodic dysmenorrhoea, and symptoms of the second half of the month; for certain menopausal conditions; for insufficient lactation.

Dosage: ½-1 gram dried fruit equivalent three times per day.

Agrimonia eupatoria, agrimony.

agrimony, Cocklebur, Stickwort, Church Steeples, *Agrimonia eupatoria* L. Fam: Rosaceae.

A perennial herb growing 30-90cm high, the erect stem bearing long spikes of flowers each 5-8mm across, bright yellow, arranged in the axil of a small cleft bract; the leaves are pinnate and stipulate; the lower leaves with 3-6 pairs of larger leaflets with 2-3 pairs of smaller leaflets in between; the fruit are enclosed in a characteristic tough capsule with a circle of hooked spines.

Habitat: throughout Britain, Europe, Asia and North America, on roadsides, wasteland, fieldsides, hedges and banks, preferring sunny positions.

Constituents: tannins, bitter principles, silica, essential oil.
Actions: astringent and haemostatic; tissue healer; diuretic.

Applications: to irritations and infections of the intestinal tract, especially in children; for gall-bladder disease associated with gastric hyperacidity; locally for ulcerated conditions and discharging skin and mucous membrane inflammations, and for conjunctival problems; urinary infections and colic.

Dosage: 1-4 grams of the dried herb equivalent three times per day.

Agropyron repens,   couch grass.

Alchemilla arvensis,   parsley piert.

Alchemilla vulgaris,   ladies' mantle.

---

alcoholism,   the condition of long-term excess alcohol intake and of the symptoms and damage associated with this habit. Consumption of alcohol must be controlled before any treatment of its effects is worthwhile, but if so allowed the **hepatic** remedies are most often effective.

---

alder buckthorn,   Frangula bark, Black Dogwood, Black Alder, Arrow-wood, *Rhammus frangula* L. Fam: Rhamnaceae.

The inner yellow bark of an erect shrub up to 6 metres in height with long upright branches with shiny brown bark and pronounced light markings (lenticels), showing a crimson layer when scraped, above the yellow inner bark; there are no thorns; the dark-green, entirely smooth leaves turn yellow or red in autumn before falling; the flowers arise from leaf axils in the upper branches, being small, greenish-white and giving way to globular berries, green turning to red and finally glossy black.

Habitat: widespread in damp woods, hedgerows, marshes and swamps in England, Wales, Europe and North America, preferring acid and light sand or peaty soils.

Constituents: **anthraquinone glycosides,** flavonoids, bitters, tannins, volatile oil, resins.

Actions: gentle purgative, cholagogue, antiparasitic.

Applications: to atonic **constipation** as short-term relief; in obstructive conditions of biliary tract; as a general blood-cleanser for chronic toxic conditions associated with bowel or digestive disturbances; as a mouth-wash for gum disease and mouth infections, and a rinse for infestations of the scalp or pubic hair; to aid in regulating disturbed bowel colonization.

Dosage: 1-2 grams of dried bark equivalent three times per day; as a laxative 2-6 grams before retiring at night.

Caution: the bark must be at least a year in storage before use; it should not be applied to constipation due to colonic tension, or for very long as a laxative.

---

alfalfa, *see* **lucerne.**

---

alkaloid, a nitrogen-containing constituent of plants, usually with potent pharmacological actions. Most plants contain some alkaloids though they do not always appear to contribute to the overall action of the herb. Being dramatically active they often catch the attention of the orthodox pharmacologist and many form the basis of allopathic drugs. Examples include morphine and the other opiate alkaloids, nicotine, quinine, ergotamine, reserpine, strychnine, mescaline, psilocybine, caffeine, ephedrine, cocaine, physostigmine, vincristine and vinblastine.

---

allergy, a hypersensitivity to one or more constituents of the environment. Most often inherited as a tendency, manifested as allergic eczema, nettle rash, hay fever, asthma or food allergies. Often an early food allergy is central and this possibility should be investigated closely; digestive functions should generally be looked at and corrected with appropriate remedies if necessary — **bitters** are often indicated. See also under specific headings for allergic conditions.

Allium sativum, garlic.

---

aloes, Curaçao or Barbados aloes, *Aloe vera* L.; Cape aloes, *A. ferox* Mill. Fam: Liliaceae.

The dried sap of the leaves of a very large succulent plant up to 3 metres in height with the large stem supporting a rosette of spine-covered leaves and an annual tall flowerstem.

Habitat: in hot dry climates of southern and eastern Africa; also in the West Indies.

Constituents: anthraquinone-related glycosides called aloins (including barbaloin), aloe-emodin, resin.

Actions: stimulating laxative; soothing and healing to the damaged tissues; uterine stimulant; anthelmintic.

Applications: to atonic constipation (combined with carminative remedies); as a local healing agent for wounds, burns, irritable rashes, stings and bites; for suppressed menstruation (but *see* **emmenogogue**).

Dosage: 120-300mg of dried sap equivalent three times per day (generally) in the form of other preparations.

Aloe vera, aloes.

---

alopecia areata, patchy baldness mainly in adolescents and young adults, of uncertain origin; spontaneous recovery is usual, although regrown hair may be lighter or white. Treatment should concentrate on improving any debilitating conditions, and diseases of teeth, gums or throat; **relaxants** may be indicated, or the problem taken as a sign of hormonal turbulence. *See also* **baldness.**

Alpinia officinarium, galanga.

---

alterative, strictly a medicine that alters the processes of metabolism so that the tissues can best deal with the functions of nutrition and elimination. The term has been largely superseded in recent times by the term 'blood-purifier' but this is no better a description for what is still an ill-understood effect. Many alteratives improve eliminations from the body and are discussed under **eliminatory remedies:** others are **hepatics, bitters** or **anti-infective.** Remedies nost often thought of as alterative include burdock, nettles, blue flag, red clover, echinacea, figwort, curled dock and cleavers. They are most often applied to toxic conditions, as manifested in chronic inflammatory states such as skin disease, arthritis and the auto-immune diseases. *See also* **detoxify.**

Althaea officinalis, marshmallow.

---

ammoniac, Ammoniacum, Gum Ammoniac, *Dorema ammonicum* G. Don. Fam: Umbelliferae.

The gum resin from the stems of a plant native to Iran; it occurs as masses or individual nodules, pale when fresh but brown when aged, breaking to expose a glossy white or pale-brown surface; the flavour is acrid, the odour characteristic.

Constituents: resin, volatile oil, salicylates.

Actions: a relaxant and peripheral vasodilator; broad-range expectorant.

Applications: to respiratory infections and for managing fever arising from such a cause (e.g., influenza); for congestive and chronic bronchitis, but may also be applied to asthmatic syndromes

Dosage: 0.3-1 gram resin equivalent three times per day.

---

anaemia, lowered levels of haemoglobin in the blood leading to a reduction in the capacity of the circulation to carry oxygen to the tissues. There are several possible causes but the most significant are excessive loss of blood, as in excessive menstrual bleeding, childbirth, gastro-intestinal disease or accident, and inadequate intake or absorption of iron. In all such cases improved dietary intake of iron is essential, either through foods or supplements. The herb parsley and green turnip tops are striking sources among the plant world.

Pernicious anaemia is not as serious a condition as it was now that the missing factor has been isolated. It requires vitamin B_{12} administration. Other anaemias may be caused by haemolytic disease or poisoning or disease of the bone marrow. Gastric and other digestive function should be examined in all cases of anaemia and treated with herbs as appropriate.

---

analgesic, pain-relieving. Notable among plants for this property is the opium poppy, and the best modern pain-relievers are still derived from this plant. Denied its use today herbalists rely on other remedies, notably gelsemium, Jamaica dogwood, Californian poppy, aconite and wild lettuce. All these plants, however, are potentially dangerous, and most are limited to professional use in the U.K. They *must* not be used without full training. All pain-relievers depress vital functions, and almost all are fatal in quantity.

Anemone pulsatilla, pasque flower.

Anethum graveolens, dill.

---

angelica, *Angelica archangelica* L. Fam: Umbelliferae.

The root or seeds of a large biennial plant, reaching over 2 metres in its second year; in its first year appears as a rosette of large bipinnate leaves on long, thick, hollow stalks much dilated at their base; in the second year a hollow fluted stem is produced surmounted by a series of umbels of small greenish-white flowers, succeeded by pale-brown oblong fruits with membranous edges, flattened on one side and convex on the other, this latter bearing three prominent ribs; the whole plant has a strong pleasant aroma.

Habitat: indigenous to the Levant but spreading to northern latitudes and entering Europe from the north, widely cultivated for its candied stems and found frequently as a naturalized escape; it prefers moist places.

Constituents: volatile oil (including phellandrene), bitter principles, tannin, resin.

Actions: warming digestive tonic; relaxing **expectorant;** antispasmodic and carminative; diuretic.

Applications: to convalescence from debilitating illnesses, especially where marked by subjective feelings of chill or cold; to improving debilitated digestive and hepatic conditions; as a component of a fever-management strategy where the condition is well entrenched; for asthmatic conditions and children's respiratory ailments.

Dosage: 1-2 grams of dried root or seed equivalent three times per day.

Angelica archangelica, angelica.

Angelica sinensis, dong quai.

---

angina pectoris, violent paroxysms of pain and pressure in the chest arising from restricted blood supply to the heart muscle; as much a functional as an organic disorder, so often directly associated with exertion and stress, passing off with rest. Arteriosclerosis of the coronary blood vessels can be assumed, producing a borderline insufficiency of supply that becomes obvious when the heart is stimulated to extra exertion'. Any heart problem will require careful professional attention. A qualified herbal practitioner may use hawthorn and/or motherwort as part of a wider regime of treatment.

---

aniseed, Anise, *Pimpinella anisum* L., Fam: Umbelliferae.

The dried ripe fruits of an annual herb of 40-60cm in height, umbelliferous in appearance with leaves varying in shape from heart-shaped to feathery; the fruit are covered with short hairs and each contain two dark seeds with light ribs; the odour and taste are characteristic.

Habitat: native to Turkey and the Levant but found growing wild as an escape in many countries.

Constituents: volatile oil (including anethole).

Actions: relaxing expectorant; carminative, antiseptic.

Applications: to bronchial infections and spasmodic coughs, specifically for tracheal irritations; to reduce the symptoms of whooping cough; to flatulence and colic and as an accompaniment for stimulating laxatives; the oil may be applied locally to scabies and lice infestations.

Dosage: 0.5-1 gram of dried fruits equivalent three times per day.

---

ankylosing spondylitis, a form of **auto-immune** disease rather like **rheumatoid arthritis** affecting particularly the spine and rib cage in young men. Can be progressively debilitating. An inherited factor is established but there are other contributory causes. The herbal practitioner will be concerned to review all possible factors, but will make particular note of any sign of infection in the urinary system or lungs, present or in the past. Treating these areas will often reduce exacerbation of the condition, sometimes considerably.

---

anodyne, a remedy that reduces pain and irritation (*see* **analgesic**).

---

anorexia, loss of appetite, an accompaniment of many, especially debilitating, diseases. A healthy sign in acute conditions like fever, but worrying if overextended. Use of **bitters** is usually indicated to both aid appetite and improve digestion overall. (*See also* **anorexia nervosa**.)

---

anorexia nervosa, a loss of appetite occurring as part of a complex disturbance of self-image and relationship with food, most often affecting girls and young women. Can be very severe. Treatment must emphasize support and care for the sufferer as a whole: herbs may be used as part of the treatment if the patient will accept them. Condurango is almost specific, but a selection of **bitters** or **relaxants** may be indicated.

---

anthelmintic, describing a remedy that produces the death or elimination of parasites from the gut. Intestinal worms were one of the most common problems in early times and many plants were used for their effect in expelling the infestation. Notable examples included wormwood, male fern, tansy, garlic, kousso, butternut and aloes, often with strong purgatives added as well. The difficulty in killing intestinal worms without harming the patient has meant, however, that skill was always required in administering anthelmintics and the task should be left entirely to trained practitioners.

Anthemis nobilis, Chamomile, Roman.

anthraquinone laxatives, laxative plants containing significant proportions of yellow substances called anthraquinone glycosides. These are absorbed across the walls of the small intestine and, 8-14 hours after ingestion, stimulate the large intestinal wall to amplified contractions and thus an increased chance of a bowel movement. Laxatives that contain these ingredients include senna pods, cascara sagrada, alder buckthorn, rhubarb root, aloes and curled dock. There is a tendency with some to cause griping, and simultaneous prescription of carminatives like fennel or dill is recommended. These laxatives should not be taken for extended periods as they numb ordinary bowel reflexes in time; they should *never* be taken where constipation is due to tension (*see* **constipation**).

antibiotic, *see* **anti-infective.**

anti-infective, a term used for those herbal remedies which may be applied to help the body withstand infections or infestations. It is used in preference to 'antiseptic' to reduce the impression that the herbs are directly active against germs or parasites themselves. In most cases it is thought that they act instead to enhance the body's own, already formidable, defences: to improve defective resistance to infection and the capacity to terminate one already present. Only a trained practitioner, however, will be able to determine when these remedies will be sufficient alone; others should not lightly discount antibiotics when an infection is established. Notable anti-infectives include echinacea, wild indigo, myrrh, raw garlic and marigold. *See also* **antiseptic.**

anti-inflammatory, description applied to any remedy that is observed to reduce inflammation or the severity of an inflammatory disease (such as arthritis). In fact such herbs appear to work more in encouraging the inflammation in its task of cleansing the area concerned than in simply suppressing the inflammatory process in the conventional sense. Some anti-inflammatories do, however, contain significant quantities of aspirin-related salicylates: they include willow bark, wintergreen, birch, meadowsweet, the poplars, and black haw; others contain constituents chemically close to steroid drugs, such as licorice, wild yam and ginseng. Notable miscellaneous anti-inflammatory remedies include lignum vitae, poke root, devil's claw, black cohosh and sarsaparilla. The majority of herbal remedies may reduce inflammations through eliminative circulatory or metabolic action: notable are celery seed, bogbean, figwort, germander, kava-kava, comfrey, dandelion, gentian, marigold, golden seal, burdock and heartsease.

antiseptic, often used to describe herbs used against infections (but *see* **anti-infective**), more strictly applied to those remedies that are directly antagonistic to pathogenic organisms on contact. Most **volatile oils** fit into this category but they rarely occur in strong enough concentrations in the whole plant to exhibit this action; the same is true for many other plant constituents in isolation, notably some **alkaloids**. In practice herbs with high proportions of **acrid** constituents and **resins** are those most likely to control micro-organisms by contact. Very high levels of **tannin** are completely antiseptic, and several plants may safely be used as wound washes for this influence. Some plants have been observed with directly anti-fungal effects, notably arbor-vitae, marigold, thyme, ivy and bittersweet.

antispasmodic, reducing spasm or tension, especially in the visceral smooth muscle, the muscle of the gut wall, bronchial tubes, bile and urinary ducts, and blood vessels. Remedies with this property are used to control functional tensions in these areas (*see* **relaxants**).

anxiety, when excessive or long-standing may be relieved by the use of herbal **relaxants,** which combine a gentle tranquillizing action with variable amount of tonifying support. Specifically supportive remedies such as damiana and oatstraw are often additionally advisable.

aperient, a mild laxative, helping to promote only a natural movement of the bowels rather than provoking them forcibly. Examples include the bulk laxatives based on agar-agar and the seaweed gums, psyllium seed and linseed, and dietary fibre; other plant remedies with gentle laxative action include rhubarb root and curled dock.

Aphanes arvensis, parsley piert.

aphrodisiac, stimulating sexual functions. An often sensationalized concept but not without validity. Adequate sexual performance is dependent on there being general well-being; successful treatment of other problems may result in transformation of a sexual problem. Several remedies are noted for a specific effect: damiana, saw palmetto, cola, yohimbe and muira-puama. For each there is some evidence to back such a claim.

Apium graveolens, celery.

appendicitis, infection and inflammation of the appendix at the base of the ascending colon. Usually of dramatic onset with severe pains in the umbilical region moving to the right lower abdomen, sensitivity over that area, constipation, often vomiting, yellow-furred tongue. Necessitates drastic treatment and should be referred to a doctor without delay. 'Grumbling appendicitis' is diagnosed more often than is justified but repeated low-grade inflammation of the appendix or associated structures is possible. Agrimony is most appropriate for this condition especially when encountered in children; other **astringents, relaxants** or **carminatives** are indicated as appropriate.

appetite, lack of, *see* **anorexia.**

arbor vitae, Tree of Life, American Cedar, *Thuja occidentalis* L. Fam: Cupressaceae.
 The leaf tips of a conical coniferous tree, reaching in its native haunts a height of up to 20 metres; the twigs appear flattened with scale-like leaves; the odour camphoraceous.

Habitat: indigenous to north-eastern North America, forming dense forests; prefers wet soil and especially stream banks; grown in gardens in Europe.

Constituents: volatile oil (including thujone), flavonoid (thujin), tannin, mucilage.

Action: stimulant to smooth muscle, particularly the bronchial muscle, the genito-urinary system, and vasculature; antiseptic; anti-inflammatory; 'stimulating alterative'.

Applications: to bronchial conditions especially with congestive heart failure or of the chronic infective type; urinary infections; as a stimulating constituent of a herbal regime for the treatment of carcinomas, especially of the chest and breasts, and psoriasis; congestive 'toxic' conditions in general; locally for vaginal infections and warts.

Dosage: 1-2 grams dried herb equivalent three times per day.

Caution: not to be used in pregnancy.

Arctium lappa, burdock.

Arctostaphylos uva-ursi, uva-ursi.

Armoracia rusticana, horseradish.

---

arnica, Leopard's Bane, Wolf's Bane, *Arnica Montana* L. Fam: Compositae.

The flowerheads of a small herbaceous perennial with a creeping underground stem giving rise to a rosette of pale ovate leaves and then, a year later, flowering stems up to 60cm high with *paired* leaves at intervals and terminating in single bright-yellow composite flowers; the plant is pleasantly aromatic.

Habitat: in mountain pastures throughout central Europe, preferring acid peaty soil.

Constituents: volatile oil, bitter principle (arnicin), vasoactive constituents of uncertain identity.

Action: stimulates the cardiovascular system on internal application, and the peripheral blood supply when externally applied; locally healing.

Applications: externally to bruises, sprains and swellings.

Dosage: the tincture BPC may be applied externally as required.

Caution; taken internally this remedy is toxic (homoeopathic preparations are extremely diluted and are thus tolerated); it should only be applied to unbroken skin and withdrawn at the first sign of dermatitis.

Arnica montana, arnica.

arrhythmia, variation from the regular rhythm of the heartbeat, including fibrillation, extrasystole and tachycardia. May be very serious but most cases merely reduce the maximum capacity of the heart in exertion and stress. Conventional heart drugs will usually have been prescribed and any herbal measure must be most carefully monitored by a professional practitioner. In practice hawthorn and/or lily-of-the-valley are most likely to be prescribed.

Artemisia absinthium, wormwood.

Artemisia abrotanum, southernwood.

Artemisia vulgaris, mugwort.

arteriosclerosis, or more strictly atherosclerosis, is sometimes referred to as 'hardening of the arteries'. It is the end result of a process of fatty infiltration and later calcification of the walls of the arteries. It is known to be associated with high levels of fats and cholesterol in the bloodstream, with smoking, with lack of exercise and high blood-pressure. If arteries to the kidneys are affected, more fluid accumulates in the body and blood-pressure will go up; the same follows after more widespread involvement of the body's arteries; if the brain is involved, mental performance may be slowed and senility hastened; if the heart, **angina** or **coronary** troubles may arise; generally the risk of **thrombosis** and other cardiovascular problems is increased. Diet should avoid fats and cholesterol and heavy drinking; smoking should be banned, and tea and coffee heavily curtailed. Exercise should be increased, under supervision if necessary. Herbalists tend to use **peripheral vasodilatory** remedies, particularly hawthorn and limeflowers, for their ability to improve circulation and oxygenation. Of these latter, garlic has notable benefits, and a long-term regime of garlic 'perles' is usually advisable.

arthritis, inflammation of a joint. A feature of many conditions but chief forms include **osteoarthritis, rheumatoid arthritis, gout,** and the degenerative **auto-immune diseases.** Approaches to each case will vary but in general the aim of herbal treatment is to improve the cleansing of these easily congested tissues. Many remedies effective in joint disease are primarily diuretic; however, the traditional approach to joint cleansing has emphasized the stimulation of circulation in the area, especially by applying **rubefacients** locally, even to the point of provoking blister formation (*see* **vesicants**). Emphasis is also put on restricting the intake of foods that are likely to contribute extra acid wastes after digestion, notably animal products and refined carbohydrates and sweets.

---

artichoke, globe, *Cynara scolymus* L. Fam: Compositae
The leaves, stem and root of a large member of the thistle family with a rosette of large, divided and toothed leaves, pale and downy on the underside, from the centre of which arises a stout stem up to 1.5 metres in height supporting the well-known globes that, if left unpicked, develop to large violet flowerheads.
Habitat: native to southern Europe but widely grown elsewhere as a vegetable.
Constituents: a bitter principle (cynarin, and sesquiterpene lactones); alkaloids; tannins; a milk-curdling enzyme (cynarase).
Actions: cholagogue; stimulating liver cell regeneration; diuretic.
Applications: to gall-bladder and biliary disease; chronic liver disease and liver impairment; some kidney disease (e.g. possibly in cases of nephrotic syndrome and albuminurea); traditionally applied for atherosclerosis and diabetes mellitus.
Dosage: 1-4 grams of the dried leaves, stem or root equivalent three times per day.

---

asafoetida, Devil's Dung, *Ferula asa-foetida* L., *F. foetida* Reg., *F. spp.* Fam. Umbelliferae.
The oleo-gum resin from the fresh roots and rhizomes of a perennial herb indigenous to Iran and western Afghanistan; the gum is found in irregular masses of agglutinated tears in a muddy grey or yellow colour, that leaves a white surface turning pink when broken; the odour is strongly onion-like; the taste is acrid.
Constituents: resin, volatile oil, gum.
Actions: antispasmodic and circulatory stimulant; calming intestinal and digestive upsets particularly; stimulating expectorant.

Applications: to colic, flatulence and dyspepsia as well as to nervous colitis and other symptoms of agitation affecting digestion; for other cases of nervous tension, insomnia, excitability, convulsions and all children's irritability; for scanty and painful menstruation in women of nervous disposition; its warming influence is prominent and suggests its use where the sufferer is susceptible to cold and colds; it is an effective stimulating expectorant for use particularly in congestive bronchial conditions. Its nauseous taste is the main limitation to wider use and it is generally given in capsule form with other remedies.

Dosage: 0.2-1 gram of resin equivalent three times per day.

Asclepias tuberosa,   pleurisy root.

---

ash,   *Fraxinus excelsior* L. Fam: Oleaceae.

The leaves and young bark of the familiar tree of temperate zones of Europe, marked out by its black buds in spring and long-stalked opposite pinnate leaves.

Constituents: glycosides ('fraxin'), flavonoids, mannite, coumarins, essential oil, tannins, resins.

Actions: laxative and diuretic; the bark was formerly used as a substitute for quinine in reducing the excesses of fever; promotes the excretion of uric acid.

Applications: to arthritic and gouty conditions where kidney and bowel function is deficient; will also directly reduce inflammation in rheumatic conditions.

Dosage: 1-2 grams of the bark or leaves equivalent three times per day.

---

asparagus,   *Asparagus officinalis* L. Fam: Liliaceae

The root of the well-known garden plant, preferably used in the fresh state.

Constituents: asparagin, saponins, rutin and other flavonoids, tannins, high levels of potassium salts.

Actions: diuretic and soothing on the urinary system, generally antispasmodic.

Applications: wherever increased flow of urine is desirable: oedema (especially arising from congestive right heart failure), urinary infections and calculi; is supportive enough on the kidneys to be applied to the diminished urine production of chronic kidney disease; will reduce the intensity of colic arising from urinary stones, and the pain arising from urinary infections.

Dosage: 20-50ml of freshly expressed juice of the fresh root three times per day.

Aspidosperma quebracho-blancho,   quebracho.

---

asthma, attacks of breathlessness brought about by spasmodic contraction of the bronchial tubes exacerbated by the secretion of a very thick, sticky mucus instead of the normal fluid phlegm. Most of the symptoms arise from an allergic process or hypersensitivity reaction taking place in the bronchial walls; treatment therefore is directed to reducing sensitivity and the exaggerated response of the bronchi. Symptomatic treatment may involve such remedies as ephedra, lobelia and jimson weed (all confined to professional practice), and grindelia, skunk cabbage, euphorbia, blood root, sundew and thyme. Relaxing **expectorants** and **antispasmodics** may find general application but the aim of the professional medical herbalist will be to find individual clues to the underlying constitutional sensitivity and to treat at the deepest background level.

---

astringent, a term denoting the binding action of many herbal remedies on mucous membranes and exposed tissues; in most cases brought about by the action of a group of constituents called **tannins** which act to 'curdle' protein molecules (like boiling an egg), a property used through the ages to make leather from animal skins. Put very simply, the action of astringent remedies is to produce a 'leather coat' on mucous or exposed surfaces, thus numbing such surfaces to irritation, checking surface inflammation, and providing an impenetrable barrier to most infective organisms and many toxins (*see* **burns** for a specific application of these properties). Such applications justify the use of astringent remedies in wound treatment, but the most widespread use is for treatment of problems of the gut wall. Traditionally astringents were applied to the management of **diarrhoea,** where the numbing and anti-inflammatory effect on the wall of the small intestine in enteritis reduces the reflex evacuation of the large bowel; a similar approach can be used to contain any inflammation or irritation of the gut wall, from **hiatus hernia, gastritis, peptic ulcers,** through to **colitis, diverticulitis** and **haemorrhoids.** Unfortunately, excessive use of tannins leads to interference in absorption of food materials (although the action is very transient in any one case, due to continuous replacement of the gut wall by regrowth and desquamation) and so their use should be short-term. Notable astringents include oak bark, catechu, rhatany root, jambul, bistort, tormentil root, witch hazel, cranesbill, and generally any part of deciduous trees. Astringency is, however, a significant feature of a very large number of herbs, and plays a notable part in the action of such as agrimony, avens, ladies' mantle, blessed thistle, blackberry leaves, eyebright, germander, bur-marigold, comfrey, white pond lily, periwinkle, golden seal, mouse-ear, plantain, stone root and sage, among others.

---

athlete's foot, a fungal infection of the skin, usually between the toes. May be treated externally with tinctures of marigold, arbor-vitae, myrrh. If infections are recurrent then investigation of the general health of the sufferer will be necessary.

Atropa belladonna, deadly nightshade.

---

auto-immune disease, an often very complex and intractable inflammatory disease brought about through the body being attacked by its own defences. The nature of the condition will depend on that part of the body attacked: classic examples include **rheumatoid arthritis, ulcerative colitis, Crohn's disease, ankylosing spondylitis,** multiple sclerosis, glomerulonephritis, **psoriasis,** polymyalgia rheumatica, pernicious anaemia, chronic **hepatitis,** systemic lupus erythematosus, many cases of thyroid disease, juvenile **diabetes mellitus;** a great many other diseases are either entirely auto-immune or have a significant auto-immune element, including **cancer** itself. Auto-immune problems are becoming more frequent in modern civilized society. Although a new threat, there is much that traditional medicines may do. Specifically there appears to be an advantage in thoroughly reviewing the whole body for signs of low-grade infections, or a history of any severe infection that might point to a residual 'brackishness': areas to look at most are lungs, urinary system and gut. There are persistent associations between sub-clinical infections and an exacerbatory factor in auto-immune disease. Appropriate **eliminative** remedies are particularly effective in removing such possible influences; beyond that the search is undertaken for any other aspect of the condition that may lend itself to a herbal approach (particular attention is paid to the liver, as concerned with regulating immunological activity in the body, *see* **liver disease**). In order to devise the best strategy a professional medical herbalist should be consulted: it is then quite possible to effect a significant improvement in many cases.

Avena sativa,   oats.

---

avens,   Herb Bennet, Benedict's Herb, Clove root, Colewort, *Geum urbanum* L. Fam: Rosaceae.

A perennial herb with erect slightly branched stems between 30 and 60cm in height, with stalked, toothed and segmented basal leaves, becoming smaller up the stem; the yellow five-petalled flowers arise at the tip of each branch, pointed sepals being visible between each pair of petals; the root is strongly aromatic with a scent reminiscent of cloves; the fruits are contained in small brown burred tassels.

Habitat: in northern temperate regions in hedgerows and woods.

Constituents: tannins, volatile oil (including eugenol), bitter principles, resin.

Actions: astringent and anti-inflammatory on exposed surfaces, with particular action on the gut wall; reputed to have additional healing capabilities as well.

Applications: to inflammatory conditions of the lower bowel (e.g., ulcerative colitis, diverticulitis); other causes of diarrhoea and any gut-wall irritation; as a gargle for sore throat and a douche for vaginal and cervical inflammations and infections.

Dosage: 1-4 grams of dried herb or root equivalent three times per day.

B

---

babies' problems,   although herbs can be extremely gentle remedies, and many are eminently suitable for correcting problems in babies and children (*see* **children's remedies**), it is obvious that special precautions are appropriate: dosage should be cut, to a quarter of adult dose or less, up to the age of two years; as far as unweaned breast-fed infants are concerned it is better to treat the mother, knowing that most of the active ingredients will pass into the milk (one can apply this principle further: many cases of infant colic can be treated by the simple expedient of cutting out cow's milk from the mother's diet, and other transmitted sensitivities are possible). For teething and other nervous irritations, many of the

relaxants are applicable, but there is often little substitute for good feeding, warmth and, above all, comfort and security.

---

backache, the herbal approach is to help reduce contributory muscle tension with **antispasmodics** where appropriate, to help correct inflammation (such as lumbago) with **anti-inflammatory** remedies, and **osteoarthritis** or other **arthritis** as relevant. In most cases rest and possibly manipulative treatment will also be necessary. Local application by massage of **rubefacient** remedies (perhaps in the form of liniments) may possibly help, and an oil made up from extractives of cramp bark and lobelia will help local muscle spasm.

---

baldness, where associated with age, due usually to hormonal changes: may possibly be ameliorated by keeping the scalp well supplied with good circulation, through regular vigorous massage or using mild **rubefacient** lotions. Excessive use of shampoos and cosmetic applications may contribute to hair loss. Rinsing or washing the hair with rosemary and/or sage infusions is beneficial. Quillaia bark in hot water makes an excellent hair cleanser. In cases of hair loss associated with disease, then such underlying conditions should be treated rather than the scalp. The loss of hair is always exacerbated by seborrheic eczema, *see* **dandruff.**

Ballota nigra, horehound, black.

---

balm, *see* **lemon balm**

---

balm of gilead, Poplar buds, *Populus gileadensis* Rouleau; also *P. balsamifera var. andicans* A Gray ('Tamacahac'). Fam: Salicaceae.
    The buds of at least two species of poplar; they are conical or pyramidal in shape, up to 25mm long, red-brown and covered with a tacky resin.
    Habitat: along streams and roadsides throughout northern North America.
    Constituents: salicin and other salicylates, oleo-resin.
    Actions: antiseptic and stimulating expectorant; gentle circulatory stimulant.
    Applications: to infections of the upper respiratory system, especially the larynx; congestive bronchial infections.

Dosage: 1-4 grams of dried buds equivalent (most used in syrup or alcohol extract) three times per day.

Note: the original, biblical balm of Gilead is the resin of a shrubby tree of the Middle East, *Commiphora ophobalsamum.*

---

balmony, Turtlebloom, Snake head, Shellflower, *Chelone glabra* L. Fam: Scrophulariaceae.

The leaves of an erect perennial herb, smooth, opposite and oblong in shape, paler on the underside with raised veins; the stem supports dense terminal spikes of slipper-like flowers, white, pink or purple; available commercially as dull leaf fragments with bitter taste.

Habitat: wet and swampy ground through eastern North America.

Constituents: not established, but including bitter principles.

Actions: digestive stimulant and gentle cholagogue; tonic; anthelmintic.

Applications: to debilitated conditions of the digestion, e.g., after febrile diseases and especially where the liver has been involved; particularly suitable for the young and elderly patient; chronic liver disease with jaundice; gallstones.

Dosage: 0.5-2 grams of dried leaf equivalent three times per day.

Baptisia tinctoria, wild indigo.

---

barberry, *Berberis vulgaris* L. Fam: Berberidaceae.

The bark of a thorned shrub with yellow wood up to 2.5 metres high, with arched and hanging branches, with clusters of alternate pale-green, stiff and toothed leaves; small yellow flowers with an unpleasant smell in elegant drooping racemes give way to small red oblong berries.

Habitat: thickets and open woods over Europe, Asia, and the northeast and west of North America; introduced to Britain.

Constituents: alkaloids (including berberine, oyacanthine, palmatine and columbamine), chelidonic acid, tannins, wax.

Actions: cholagogue and hepatic stimulant; stimulating digestive tonic.

Applications: to gallstones and biliary infections; to debilitated conditions marked by poor digestive function and a history of dietary or alcohol abuse, or excessive exposure to drugs, chemicals or industrial pollutants; splenic enlargement; to leishmaniasis and malaria.

Dosage: 0.5-2 grams of dried bark equivalent three times per day.

Caution: this remedy must be avoided in pregnancy and in excessive doses.

Barosma betulina, buchu.

---

bayberry, Waxberry, Candleberry, Wax myrtle, *Myrica cerifera* L. Fam: Myricaceae.

The root bark of a shrub 0.6 to 2.5 metres high with smooth grey bark and smooth ovate pointed leaves that are slightly toothed and often downy underneath; the waxy, bluish-white berries are produced in clusters on the flowering shoots; the root bark is reddish to brown and occurs commercially in flat pieces, with short fracture though slightly fibrous on the inner side, sweet, tickling aromatic odour and bitter astringent taste.

Habitat: native to the woods and marshes of eastern North America.

Constituents: tannins, resin (myrinic acid), volatile oil.

Actions: circulatory stimulant; locally astringent; tonic.

Applications: to looseness, inflammation and infection of the bowels; as a component (especially with cayenne or ginger) of warming and sustaining treatments for use in febrile, cachexic and chronically inflamed conditions; for excessive menstrual bleeding and uterine discharge, both systemically and locally as a douche; as a gargle for throat infections, and topically for slow-healing wounds and ulcers.

Dosage: 0.5-2 grams of dried root equivalent three times per day.

---

bearberry, *see* **uva-ursi.**

---

bed-wetting, or enuresis, is considered a medical problem when it occurs regularly in someone over the age of five years, either as a primary problem (i.e., where control has never developed) or as 'onset enuresis' (where the problem has started after a period of normal control). In both cases the problem has its origin mostly in, often well-disguised, anxiety. The best approach is to combine appropriate training measures with herbal **relaxants,** notably cramp bark, with specific remedies such as corn silk, horsetail, or periwinkle, and to have attention to any event that may be producing undue anxiety in the child concerned.

Berberis aquifolium, oregon grape.

Berberis vulgaris, barberry.

---

beth root, Birth root, Wake robin, *Trillium erectum* L., *T. pendulum* Willd. Fam: Liliaceae.

The rhizone and roots of a stout erect perennial herb with a simple stem bearing a whorl of three broad rhombic pointed leaves and terminating in a large terminal flower with six petals, pruple or pale-green or palebrown; the rhizone is obtained as hard fragments, transversely ringed and with numerous fibrous rootlets.

Habitat: rich woodland in central and western states of the U.S.A.

Constituents: steroidal saponins (including trillarin), steroidal glycoside, tannins, fixed oil.

Actions: antihaemorrhagic, with particular action on the female reproductive system, astringent.

Applications: to heavy menstrual bleeding; as a palliative remedy for blood loss from urinary tract and lungs; to checking discharge from the womb, and to preventing complications in labour; applied locally as a douche for vaginal and cervical problems.

Dosage: 0.5-2 grams of dried rhizome and root equivalent three times per day.

Betonica officinalis, betony.

---

betony, Wood Betony, Bishopswort, *Betonica officinalis* L., *Stachys betonica* Benth. Fam: Labiatae.

A perennial herb up to 30-60cm with downy, crenated, oblong leaves and dense whorls of red-purple flowers in close terminal heads, each above a lanceolate bract.

Habitat: woods and thickets over Britain and Europe except in the north.

Constituents: alkaloids (including betonicine, stachydrine, trigonelline); tannins.

Actions: tonifying circulatory stimulant for the cerebral and head area; relaxant; bitter stimulant to digestion (in large doses emetic and cathartic); astringent.

Applications: to headaches particularly associated with debility and/or nervous tension; to sinus and other catarrhal congestion in the head; neuralgias; gastritis and the poor digestion of debility.

Dosage: 1-4 grams of dried herb equivalent three times per day.

Betula alba et spp, birch.

Bidens tripartita, bur-marigold.

Bilious attacks, *see* **gastritis** *and* **migraine.**

---

birch, silver, White birch, paper birch, *Betula alba* L., *B. pendula* Roth., *B. verrucosa* Ehrh. Fam: Betulaceae.

A familiar tree recognized for its silvery-white bark, peeling off in layers, and its slender drooping branches; the leaves are broadly ovate, toothed and tapering to a fine point, with minute glandular dots when young; the male catkins are drooping, 2-5cm long, the female up to 15cm long. The young leaves, bark, sap and leaf buds are all used medicinally.

Habitat: in woodlands throughout the whole northern hemisphere.

Constituents: saponins, volatile oil (including the camphor-like betulin), resin, flavonoids, tannins, bitter principle.

Actions: anti-inflammatory, diuretic; cholagogue, diaphoretic.

Applications: to rheumatic and arthritic conditions, especially where kidney functions appear to need support; to the active phases of rheumatic or other auto-immune illnesses, especially where associated with fever or serum sickness; oedematous states; urinary infections and calculi.

Dosage: 1-4 grams of dried leaves, bark or buds equivalent or 10-20ml of sap preserved with 20 per cent alcohol three times per day.

---

birth root, *see* **beth root.**

---

bistort, Adderwort, English Serpentary, Snakeweed, *Polygonum bistorta* L. Fam: Polygonaceae.

The root of a perennial plant that gives rise to simply erect stalks up to 60cm high, with few almost sessile leaves, ending in a dense spike of pink or red flowers 2-5cm long in total; basal leaves are slender and up to 15cm long; the root is S-shaped, dark to red-brown on the outside, light red-brown internally.

Habitat: moist ground mainly in mountain pastures or higher ground in Europe, central Asia and west of the Rockies in North America; in Britain found mostly in northern England and southern Scotland.

Constituents: tannins.

Actions: astringent and demulcent.

Applications: to enteric inflammation and diarrhoea; colitis and diverticulitis; as a mouthwash for stomatitis and gum disease; as a douche for vaginal and cervical inflammation and erosion; as a gargle for throat infections.

Dosage: 0.5-2 grams of dried root three times per day.

---

bitters, plants with a prominently bitter taste, due to the presence of a variety of chemical constituents including **volatile oils, alkaloids,** sesquiterpene lactones all termed 'bitter principles'. The taste of bitterness is an extremely common feature of many herbal remedies, and it is thus of some importance that this taste has a major pharmacological action. Essentially the action of bitter substances is mediated by the bitter-sensitive taste buds in the mouth: these do more than simply signify the taste of food or medicine, and are actually connected neurally in such a way that their stimulation leads to the release from the gut wall into the bloodstream of a hormone called gastrin, among other probable responses. The action in the body of gastrin has been reasonably well charted and accords closely with the claims made for the action of bitter herbs. These claims are ambitious, but well supported. Bitters (a) stimulate the appetite, and thus are applied where lack of appetite or **anorexia** is a feature of any condition; (b) increase the flow of digestive juices, and are thus indicated in sluggish **dyspepsia,** to reduce the risk of enteric infections, to reduce fermentation of gut contents in **fever management,** to reduce the antigencity of proteins in the food as a cause of **food allergies,** and generally to improve the micro-environment of the gut even in problems of the lower intestines; (c) increase bile flow and dilution, so reducing the chance of **gall-bladder disease,** and in effect acting to improve the self-cleansing reparative ability of the liver, so finding application in a wide range of **liver disease;** (d) regulate the secretion of insulin and glucagon by the endocrine pancreas, so having an important application to **hypoglycaemia** and late-onset **diabetes** (a genuine two-handed effect on these contradictory symptoms can be explained: an example of an **adaptogenic** action); (e) stimulate repair of the gut wall lining, so that bitters are not necessarily contra-indicated in **(peptic) ulcers,** and other inflammatory or erosive conditions.

In short the action of bitters can be seen to enhance the whole upper digestive function, and to improve assimilation of nutrients into the system. In traditional medicine, this property was extremely highly regarded, as leading to a real tonic improvement in health in even the most debilitated circumstances (the term **tonic,** usually denotes a bitter medicine); bitters were also seen to be 'cooling', reducing the heat of fever by switching blood flow to the breakdown of food, and reducing toxin reabsorption in such conditions, but in a more general way improving nourishment at the expense of circulatory 'heat'. In this sense one thus tends to prescribe bitters in 'hot' conditions, i.e., where the patient feels the heat too much, does not notice cold, where the condition is improved by the application of cold packs or cool air, where there is a thirst for cold drinks, where the tongue is dry, red and its coating tends to yellow, where the complexion is dark or flushed, and where there is nervous agitation, restlessness and tension. The bitter option is one of the most central choices facing the herbalist.

A great many herbs have notable bitter tastes (and it follows from the above that it is the taste that matters — the bitter effect is completely lost unless one *tastes* the bitter, and the intensity of the effect is in direct proportion to the strength of the taste); however, notable bitters include the following: gentian, wormwood, calumba, celandine, barberry, balmony, centaury, chicory, quassia, cinchona, Oregon grape, condurango, boldo, buckbean, chiretta, hops, white horehound, mugwort, southernwood, willow, germander, blessed thistle, gotu kola and quebracho.

---

bittersweet, Woody nightshade, Dulcamara, Felonwood, *Solanum dulcamara* L. Fam: Solanaceae.

A shrubby herb sending off climbing and rambling branches with stalked ovate, smooth or downy leaves 5-8cm long, sometimes divided into lobes; small blue flowers with marked yellow anthers in loose cymes often coexist with the red or black berries; the 2-3 year-old stems are the part most used in medicine.

Habitat: in moist and shady hedges and thickets over Britain and Europe.

Constituents: alkaloids (including solasodine, soladulcidine, solanine, solamarine); saponins ('dulcamarin'); tannin; resin.

Actions: helping to mitigate inflammation in chronic degenerative diseases; stimulating expectorant; possible primary action on liver functions; diuretic.

Applications: to inflammatory degenerative diseases such as rheumatoid conditions, psoriasis, eczema, especially when these are associated with bronchial or pulmonary congestion or liver debility; to chronic bronchitis; chronic liver inflammation.

Caution: although not as toxic as other members of this genus this plant has quite a potent action on the body; it should not be used by those not trained in using herbs; possible side effects are nausea, vertigo and palpitations.

Dosage: 0.5-2 grams of dried twigs equivalent three times per day.

---

blackberry leaves, Bramble leaves, *Rubus fructicosus* L. Fam: Rosaceae.

The leaves of a very common rambling shrub; they are large and coarse with 2-5 ovate, toothed leaflets, with midribs and stalks armed with small hooked prickles.

Habitat: widespread around the world in hedgerows and waste places everywhere.

Constituents: tannins, flavonoids.

Actions: astringent and healing.

Applications: to gum disease, throat infections and inflammations, mouth ulcers, as a mouthwash and gargle.

Dosage: 1-4 grams of dried herb equivalent three times per day.

---

black cohosh, Black snakeroot, Rattleroot, *Cimicifuga racemosa* Nutt. Fam: Ranunculaceae.

The rhizome and roots of a tall perennial with slender stem giving rise to occasional sprays of broad, sharply-lobed leaves and ending in terminal spikes of creamy-white flowers; the rhizome is black on the outside, bearing short, upright branches ending in a cup-shaped scar, and underneath are many long brittle roots; internally white to brown and waxy; the taste is bitter and acrid.

Habitat: woods and higher ground throughout northern and eastern North America.

Constituents: resin (cimicifugin), bitter glycoside (racemosin), salicylates, tannin, oestrogenic principle, acrid principle (ranunculin, converting to anemonin).

Actions: antispasmodic and alterative; tonic; vasodilator and diaphoretic.

Applications: muscular rheumatism, neuralgias, muscle cramps, myalgia; any inflammatory condition associated with spasm or tension; dysmenorrhoea of the spasmodic type and uterine discharges.

Dosage: 0.2-1 gram of dried rhizome equivalent three times per day.

Caution: high doses of black cohosh are potentially dangeous; they are likely to produce vertigo and visual and nervous disturbances; the plant must not be used during pregnancy; its use by the untrained in general is to be discouraged.

---

black haw, Sweet viburnum, *Viburnum prunifolium* L. Fam: Caprifoliaceae.

The root bark of a shrubby tree with pointed finely-toothed leaves on long slender stalks and sessile cymes of small white flowers giving way to bluish-black fruit; the short-pointed leaf buds are a notable feature over winter; the bark is available commercially in irregular pieces, greyish on the outside, reddish-brown on the inner surface with a bitter and astringent taste, and a slight valerian-like odour.

Habitat: central and southern North America.

Constituents: Bitter principle (viburnin), triterpenoid saponins, salicosides, resin, valeric acid, tannin, arbutin, coumarins.

Actions: having an astringent and antispasmodic effect on the female reproductive system.

Applications: to excessive menstrual flow, especially around menopause; spasmodic dysmenorrhoea, threatened miscarriage; vaginal and cervical discharges.

Dosage: 2-4 grams of dried bark equivalent three times per day.

---

black root, Culver's root, *Veronicastrum virginicum* (L) Farwell, *Leptandra virginica* (L) Nutt., *Veronica virginica* Tourn. Fam: Scrophulariaceae.

The rhizome and roots of a tall perennial herb up to 1.5 metres high with a simple erect stem producing at intervals whorls of 4-7 lanceolate, finely-toothed leaves on short stalks, and terminating in a long spike of white flowers.

Habitat: throughout the U.S.A. except the far west, though frequently cultivated around the world.

Constituents: bitter principle (leptandrin), volatile oil, saponin and phytosterols, glycoside (resembling senegin), tannins, resin.

Actions: gentle hepatic tonic with mild laxative properties.

Applications: to chronic congestive conditions of the digestion and bowel.

Dosage: 0.5-4 gram rhizome equivalent three times per day.

---

bladder problems, *see* **urinary infections, urinary stones.**

---

bladderwrack, *see* **kelp.**

---

blessed thistle, Holy thistle, *Cnicus benedictus* L., *Carduus benedictus* Steud. Fam: Compositae.

An annual thistle-like herb growing up to 40cm high with a terminal of creamy yellow composite flowers surrounded by a spiny calyx; the leaves are long and slender, sharply toothed and spiny.

Habitat: Sunny, stony and waste places in southern Europe and western Asia; found only sporadically in Britain and North America.

Constituents: bitter glycosides (including cnicin), alkaloids, volatile oil, tannins, mucilage, resin.

Actions: bitter digestive stimulant; astringent; diaphoretic.

Applications: to anorexia and sluggish digestion, especially of fevers and when there is inflammation or infection of the digestive tract.

Dosage: 1-3 grams of dried herb equivalent three times per day.

---

blood root,   Red root, Indian paint, *Sanguinaria canadensis* L. Fam: Papaveraceae.

The rhizome of a small perennial plant with kidney-shaped leaves arising directly from buds on the rootstock, with reticular veining, and greyish-green downy surface; the single naked flower stem bears a white double flower; the rhizome is dark reddish with a strong acrid and bitter taste.

Habitat: in rich open broadleaved woodland through the eastern half of North America.

Constituents: alkaloids (including sanguinarine, protopine), red resin.

Actions: a strong expectorant (emetic in large doses); cathartic; circulatory stimulant; uterine stimulant.

Applications: to infections of the respiratory tract (formerly used for severe infections as an emetic), particularly in debilated and cold conditions; locally as a snuff for nasal polyps, and for local inflammations and infections of the skin, e.g., warts.

Dosage: 0.05-0.5 grams of dried rhizome equivalent three times a day.

Caution: this plant is poisonous in large doses and should only be used by trained practitioners. It must not be used during pregnancy and lactation.

---

blue cohosh,   Papoose root, Squaw root, Blue ginseng, *Caulophyllum thalictroides* (L) Mich. Fam: Berberidaceae.

The rhizome and roots of a perennial plant up to 1 metre high with large three-lobed leaves and racemes of small yellow-green flowers; the rhizome is hard and knotted with masses of fibrous roots below and large cup-shaped scars above; with a sweet-bitter taste that becomes acrid.

Habitat: in moist rich ground in eastern North America.

Constituents: steroidal saponin (caulosapogenin), alkaloids (including magnoflorine, cytisine, laburnine).

Actions: antispasmodic, particularly for the female reproductive system; tonic effect on uterus and Fallopian tubes.

Applications: to dysmenorrhoea, especially that commencing with the menstrual flow, and occurring in adolescence; to functional amenorrhoea; to most pains and spasms of the menstrual cycle, of menopause, and to alleviate those of pelvic inflammation, fibroids, etc.; for the pains of labour and after parturition.

Dosage: 0.2-1 gram of dried rhizome equivalent three times per day.

Caution: this remedy should not be used in pregnancy until labour has commenced.

---

blue flag, *Iris versicolor* L. and *I. caroliniana* Watson. Fam: Iridaceae.

The rhizome of a perennial herb of the Iris family with large blue flowers with yellow and white markings at the base of the sepals; the dried rhizome is cylindrical or flattened, externally greyish, internally reddish-brown, with annular joints, cup-shaped stem scars, ring-shaped leaf scars and rootscars on the undersurface.

Habitat: wetlands in eastern and central North America; imported as an ornamental to many parts of the world.

Constituents: oleoresin (including isophthalic acid), salicylates, alkaloid, tannins.

Actions: circulatory and lymphatic stimulant; cholagogue and laxative; diuretic.

Applications: skin conditions, especially where associated with bowel and hepatic disturbances or strain and/or poor or congestive circulation.

Dosage: 0.5-2 grams of dried rhizome equivalent three times per day.

Caution: this remedy may irritate the digestion in some cases.

---

boils, local inflammation of the hair roots due to staphylococcal infection; most often in areas of friction. Most likely in debility and after over-eating or excessive alcohol consumption but, if frequent, may denote kidney disease or diabetes, so should be checked in this case. It is inadvisable to lance or handle boils, as infection is easily spread and the body can deal internally with any pus with ease. Provided other serious predisposing factors have been excluded, the use of **eliminatives,** especially echinacea and burdock is to be recommended. A cluster of boils is referred to as a carbuncle.

---

boldo, *Peumus boldo* Mol. Fam: Monimiaceae.

The leaves of an evergreen shrubby tree up to 6 metres high; they are glossy, leathery, 3-7cm long, 2-4cm broad, pale green above, even paler, to grey below, with prominent veins; the surface on the upper side is covered with minute papillae; there is a strong characteristic odour, aromatic and spicy.

Habitat: on dry sunny slopes in lightly wooded country in Chile.

Constituents: volatile oil, alkaloids (including boldine), glycoside (boldoglucin), resin, tannins.

Actions: cholagogue and bitter digestive stimulant; analgesic; urinary antiseptic.

Applications: gallstones, gall-bladder infection and biliary colic or other hepatic-related pain; urinary infections.

Dosage: 0.06-0.2 gram of dried leaves equivalent three times per day.

---

boneset, Feverwort, Thoroughwort, *Eupatorium perfoliatum* L. Fam: Compositae.

A perennial herb reaching 1.5 metres in height with a stout hairy stem bearing opposite pointed leaves united at the base (so as to seem 'perforated' by the stem), finely-toothed, rough above, downy and resinous below; the terminal flower clusters are white and reminiscent of the yarrow.

Habitat: in damp pastures and wet ground throughout eastern North America.

Constituents: volatile oils, glycoside (eupatorin).

Actions: peripheral vasodilator and diaphoretic; cholagogue; gentle laxative; antispasmodic.

Applications: as part of a fever-management strategy, providing an excellent diffusion of heat out of the body; particularly useful for respiratory sources of fever, such as influenza; for catarrhal conditions generally; for biliousness and constipation; any conditions exacerbated by damp; for skin disease linked to digestive and hepatic disorders; for night sweats.

Dosage: 1-3 grams of dried herb equivalent three times a day.

---

breast problems, as a glandular tissue the breast is prone to a variety of inflammatory and degenerative problems, from simple fibrous changes, through 'chronic cystic mastitis', fat necrosis, cysts, papilloma, to carcinoma in its many forms. All may produce a mix of lumpiness, pain, swelling and lymphatic enlargement so they will have to be expertly diagnosed. A general herbal approach can be had to most cases, using specific **alteratives** and **eliminatives** such as sweet violet, arbor-vitae, marigold, red clover and wild thyme. There may be a hormonal factor for the qualified practitioner to prescribe for, and other wider factors will have to be taken into account if present. Acute mastitis, found occasionally in lactating mothers, can be treated with soothing poultices, and internally with marigold, garlic and echinacea: if these are unable to check the condition quickly, tetracyclines may have to be prescribed to prevent abscess formation, the breast should be regularly pumped clear. If cancer is diagnosed usual considerations apply (*see* **cancer**).

---

bronchiectasis, the breaking down of lung tissue after chronic bronchitis or other lung disease, to leave large cavities lined by bronchiolar mucous membrane secreting quantities of mucus that is trapped in the cavities: the lack of breathing capacity and the stagnant conditions that develop are very debilitating. Continuous removal of congestion is recommended with postural drainage techniques and **stimulating expectorants;** in other ways the treatment is the same as for chronic bronchitis.

---

bronchitis, acute or chronic inflammation of the mucous membranes of the airways in the lung. A major problem, and responsible for much ill health especially in later life. The aim of herbal treatment is to promote the expectoration of congested mucus in the first instance, and this is accomplished with garlic (preferably raw) and the **stimulating expectorants.** The background weakness is treated with warming remedies such as angelica root, cinnamon, ginger, horseradish and cayenne, and these should be used regularly during any cold or damp conditions. It is also important to attend to other predisposing weaknesses, especially in circulation and digestion. Smoking and excessive alcohol, caffeine and refined carbohydrate consumption should be banned, and milk products should be limited.

---

broom, *Sarothamnus scoparius* (L) Koch. Fam: Papilionaceae.
The tips of a shrub 90-200 cm tall with smooth, long, erect, green wiry branches with five prominent angles in cross-section; lower leaves are shortly-stalked with three small ovate leaflets; upper leaves sessile and often singular; bright broad-petalled yellow, solitary or paired flowers arise out of old leaf axils giving way to long flat pods 2-5cm long, smooth on the sides but with hairy edges.
Habitat: on dry hilly areas in Britain, west Europe up to Scandinavia.
Constituents: alkaloids (including sparteine and genisteine), flavonoids (including scoparin), volatile oil, tannin.
Actions: peripheral vasoconstrictor; cardioactive; diuretic.
Applications: to palpitation, arrythmias and heart failure especially when

associated with low blood-pressure; to oedema associated with heart failure; to shock; to excessive blood loss at menstruation.

Dosage: 2-4 grams of dried tips equivalent three times per day.

Caution: the applications of this plant make it inappropriate for non-professional use; it must not be used in high blood-pressure and should not be applied in pregnancy.

Bryonia alba et spp,   bryony, white.

---

bryony, white,   Mandragora, English mandrake, Wild vine, *Bryonia alba* L., *Bryonia dioica* Jacquin. Fam: Cucurbitaceae.

The root of a perennial plant with very long annual climbing stems with spiral tendrils and leaves deeply cut into 5-7 broad angular and roughly-toothed lobes; the rootstock is thick and tuberous; the flowers are unisexual, the male's pale yellow, about 1cm across in stalked clusters, the female's in pairs, much smaller, giving rise to yellow and orange berries; the whole plant yields a foetid acrid juice when cut.

Habitat: in hedges and thickets in southern England and central and southern Europe.

Constituents: triterpenoid bitters (cucurbitacins), alkaloids (including bryonicine), phytosterols, volatile oil, tannins.

Actions: powerful purgative with toxic but possible anti-tumour activities; expectorant; vermifuge; diaphoretic; emetic in large doses.

Applications: for congestive bronchial and pulmonary conditions; for rheumatic conditions; locally for muscular, joint and pulmonary inflammations.

Dosage: 0.1-0.5 gram of dried root equivalent three times per day.

Caution: this remedy is toxic in large dosage and is not recommended for use by untrained persons; it must never be used in pregnancy.

---

buchu,   Bucco, *Agathosma betulina* (Berg) Pillans; *Barosma betulina* (Bert and Wendl) Fam: Rutaceae.

The leaves of a shrub up to 2 metres in height; the leaves are 1-2cm long, with a broad tip converging to a very short stem; bright-to-yellowish-green, darker above than below, with papillae on the upper surface marking the presence of oil glands, and very wrinkled on the lower surface; the leaves are smooth and shiny and very brittle when dry; the odour is pronounced and reminiscent of blackcurrant.

Habitat: the Cape province of South Africa.

Constituents: volatile oil (including diosphenol, limonene, menthol and camphor); glycoside (barosmin or diosmin); flavonoids; resin.
Actions: urinary antiseptic.
Applications: to all urinary and prostatic infections (one of the most efficient of all such remedies).
Dosage: 0.5-2 grams of dried leaves equivalent three times per day.

---

buckbean, Bogbean, Marsh trefoil, *Menyanthes trifoliata* L. Fam: Menyanthaceae.
An aquatic herb with a creeping rootstock and densely matted roots with a short creeping or floating stem; there are dense tufts of leaves each with long sheathed stalks and consisting of three oblong leaflets; flowers are white, tipped with red, in racemes on long stalks from each tuft of leaves.
Habitat: in bogs and shallow ponds through Britain, Europe, central Asia and North America.
Constituents: bitter glycosides (including loganin and foliamenthin), alkaloids (including gentianine), saponin, flavonoids, essential oil, coumarin (scopoletin).
Actions: bitter digestive stimulant and stimulating laxative; anti-inflammatory; diuretic.
Applications: rheumatoid arthritis associated with digestive and other debility; similar application to other chronic inflammatory conditions and auto-immune diseases.
Dosage: 0.5-2 grams of dried leaves equivalent three times per day.

---

buckwheat, *Fagopyrum esculentum* Moench. Fam: Polygonaceae.
An erect annual plant with green or red smooth stems giving off arrow-shaped or heart-shaped leaves, pale-green and soft, and spreading panicles of white-to-pink flowers, lightly perfumed and very attractive to bees; the hard nut is pyramidal in shape.
Habitat: native to Central Asia but cultivated and naturalized elsewhere, especially in North America.
Constituents: flavonoid glycosides (notably rutin).
Actions: toning and repairing blood vessel walls; vasodilatory.
Applications: to hypertension accompanied by capillary fragility and petechiae; frostbite and chilblains; capillary haemorrhages; retinal haemorrhage; radiation damage.
Dosage: 2-5 grams of dried herb equivalent three times per day.

Buerger's disease, or *thromboangiitis obliterans*, is an inflammatory condition of the arteries, mainly of the legs, marked by pain and pallor and later by ulceration and even gangrene. It is made worse by smoking but otherwise its origin is not well known. Herbal remedies that may help include hawthorn, angelica and wild yam. *See also* **Raynaud's disease.**

---

bulimia nervosa, bouts of excessive eating often followed by self-induced vomiting; generally conducted in secret as part of a syndrome that usually alternates with, and is related to, **anorexia nervosa.** Similar approaches for treatment apply, and the use of **bitters** need not be avoided.

---

burdock, Beggar's buttons, Bardane, Thorny burr, *Arctium lappa* L. Fam: Compositae.

The root and possibly leaves of a substantial biennial plant up to 2 metres in height, with very large ovate-cordate leaves up to 50cm across forming a rosette at ground level, with smaller versions growing up the thick flowering stem; the flowers are borne in clusters at the top of the stem, globular in shape and covered with a dense array of stiff hooked bracts that cling to clothes on contact; the long root runs straight down as much as a metre into the subsoil; there are several similar species of burdock and in practice the herbalist has failed to distinguish between them.

Habitat: on roadsides and waste places and around field borders throughout Britain, Europe and North America.

Constituents: bitter glycosides (including arctiopicrin), flavonoids, tannin, volatile oil, antibiotic substances (especially in the fresh sample), resin and mucilage, inulin.

Actions: a general alterative remedy appearing to exert a cleansing effect on the tissues as such; diuretic; mild laxative.

Applications: to toxic conditions resulting in skin disease, boils and sores, and other inflammatory conditions; for eczema especially when in a dry and scaling phase.

Dosage: 1-6 grams of dried root or leaf equivalent three times per day.

Caution: excessive use of this remedy may precipitate a symptomatic crisis in severely toxic conditions or where eliminatory channels are deficient: it is recommended that dosage starts cautiously, working up as appropriate.

---

bur-marigold, Water Agrimony, *Bidens tripartita* L. Fam: Compositae.

A stout, erect annual herb 30-60cm high with spreading branches and serrated leaves cut into 3-5 lanceolate segments; terminal yellow hemispherical flowerheads with tubular florets up to 3cm in diameter. *Habitat:* in wet ditches and marshes throughout Britain, Europe, Asia and North America. *Constituents:* tannins and other astringent principles, volatile oil. *Actions:* antihaemorrhagic and locally and systemically astringent. *Applications:* to control bleeding in the urinary system; to provide a healing influence to peptic and lower bowel ulceration and inflammation. *Dosage:* 1-4 grams of dried plant equivalent three times per day. **Caution:** all these indications demand expert diagnostic attention: this plant should not be used alone.

---

burnet, greater, Garden burnet, *Sanguisorba officinalis* L. Fam: Rosaceae.

An erect, smooth perennial herb around 60cm in height; a perennial rootstock gives rise to segmented ovate toothed leaves and flowering stems divided at the top into 3-4 long stems each terminated by a single head of crowded purple flowers. *Habitat:* in moist (especially mountain) meadows over England, North America and Europe. *Constituents:* tannin, flavonoids, volatile oil. *Actions:* astringent. *Applications:* to inflammations of the gut wall, such as might provoke diarrhoea. *Dosage:* 2-6 grams of dried herb equivalent three times per day.

---

burns, cases where the skin is not broken should be treated immediately by immersing in cold water: provided blisters do not form, relief may be had by applying an oil made by steeping St John's wort flowers in sunflower oil in sunlight for two weeks (until bright red liquid can be collected); if blisters form or the skin is broken, refer for medical treatment immediately; in an entirely first-aid situation, septicaemia may be prevented and healing encouraged by bathing the wound in a very strong solution of **tannins** (ideal sources are oak bark or galls or, in emergency, the bark of most deciduous trees, or even household tea in very high concentration), this to be repeated frequently until a protective 'eschar' is formed — in effect a temporary 'skin'.

---

butternut, White walnut, Oilnut, *Juglans cinerea* L. Fam: Juglandaceae

The bark of a tree up to 25 metres in height with grey, relatively smooth bark; the leaves are large and pinnate, divided into 11-19 pointed and toothed leaflets; there are drooping racemes or catkins of separate male and female flowers.

Habitat: in rich and rocky woods throughout North America.

Constituents: a naphthaquinone (juglone), tannin, essential oils.

Actions: stimulating laxative; cholagogue.

Applications: atonic constipation; to stimulate liver function in congestive or sluggish digestive disorders; to chronic or acute skin disease associated with bowel and/or liver torpor.

Dosage: 1-5 grams of dried bark equivalent three times per day.

C

cactus flowers, *Opuntia spp.* Fam: Cactaceae.

The flowers of several species of cactus, obtained commercially as pale light heads 3cm long and 1.5cm in diameter, with packed petals, with short sepals on the outside, enclosing a lobed stigma and a mass of stamens.

Habitat: Mexico.

Actions: Astringent.

Applications: irritation of the bowel, with diarrhoea or looseness; benign prostatic hypertrophy.

Dosage: 0.3-1 gram of dried flowers equivalent three times per day.

calculi, *see* **urinary stones, gallstones.**

calendula, *see* **marigold.**

Calendula officinalis, marigold.

Calluna vulgaris, heather flowers.

---

calumba, Colombo, *Jateorhiza palmata* (Lam) Miers. Fam: Menispermaceae.

The root of a perennial climbing plant with small inconspicuous dioecious flowers; the root is obtained in transverse slices 2-8cm in diameter and 3-12cm thick, with pronounced dark cambium separating a yellow outer and grey inner region; the taste is bitter.

Habitat: forest regions of East Africa and Mozambique

Constituents: alkaloids (including calumbamine, jateorhizine, palmatine, berberine, columbin); bitter glycosides; volatile oil.

Actions: bitter digestive stimulant with carminative action.

Applications: to lack of appetite and digestive weakness, particularly in fevers and afterwards; flatulence, intestinal colic and irritation.

Dosage: 0.3-1 gram of dried root equivalent three times per day.

---

cancer, like other equally valid gentle approaches to this condition, herbalism is less concerned with attacking the specific tumour than with helping as far as possible the body's own formidable fighting defences (which are responsible for eliminating some 10,000 malignant cells that are reckoned to develop on average every day of our lives). Thus, specific recognition and targeting of a tumour is less important than developing a general strategy which can be applied with individual variations to promoting health. In practice those most accomplished at applying herbs towards cancer treatment (naturopathic clinics in Europe) do so as part of a dietary, hydrotherapeutic, and counselling regime, and these features should all contribute, along with any other that promises to improve vitality. The herbal strategy is above all to initiate a thorough cleansing programme, using **eliminative** remedies, often with some vigour (depending on the strength of the patient); favoured examples of the breed are violet (sweet), red clover, arbor-vitae, marigold, cleavers and burdock, but almost any of the eliminative or **alterative** remedies may have an application; this process is maintained for as long as necessary, but it should be progressively augmented by a more restorative regime, using such remedies as will improve and maintain normal vital functions, e.g., **bitters** for digestive and liver functions, **circulatory stimulants,** and **nervous restoratives; anti-infective** and **lymphatic** remedies may help specifically to improve the body's defences. All such applications must of course be carefully considered, especially when chemotherapy or radiotherapy is contemplated, and it is strongly recommended that only qualified practitioners make such decisions.

Capsella bursa-pastoris, shepherd's purse.

Capsicum minimum et spp, cayenne.

---

caraway, *Carum carvi* L. Fam: Umbelliferae.
The seeds of a biennial plant with tap root and erect branched stem up
to 60cm high with long pinnate leaves divided into several paired linear
segments, themselves sometimes pinnate, and with long sheathed stalks;
the seeds are long, usually curved, with prominent ribs and characteristic
taste and odour.
Habitat: in moist meadows in Europe and Central Asia, rarer in the
West but naturalized in parts of Britain and North America.
Constituents: volatile oil (including carvone and limonene), fatty oil,
tannin.
Actions: gently stimulating expectorant; carminative; antispasmodic.
Applications: to colic and flatulence and intestinal overactivity;
congestive bronchitis and colds on the chest.
Dosage: 0.5-2 grams dried seeds equivalent three times per day.

---

carbuncles, *see* **boils.**

---

cardamom, *Elettaria cardamomum* Maton. Fam: Zingiberaceae.
The seeds of a large reed-like plant with flowering stems extending
horizontally along the ground, bearing loose racemes of small yellowish
flowers with purple tips; the fruits are 0.5-1cm long, pale yellowish-grey,
triangular in cross-section; each contains 3-5 cells with two seeds in each
cell; each seed is a dark, reddish-brown, oblong and angular; the whole
has a strong, characteristic odour, and a strong taste.
Habitat: Sri Lanka, Malabar coast and South-East Asia.
Constituents: volatile oil (including terpenyl acetate, limonene, cineole,
sabinene, p-cymene).
Actions: carminative; digestive stimulant; circulatory stimulant.
Applications: to flatulence and colic; digestive atony, especially when
accompanied by sensations of cold; as an accompaniment to laxatives and
bitter digestive stimulants.

Dosage: 0.5-2 grams of dried seeds equivalent three times per day.

---

cardioactive, remedies that have a noticeable action on heart function, notably applied to the foxglove-derived glycosides that are the basis of conventional treatment for heart-failure and arrhythmias; this action is to stabilize the excitability of the heart muscle and to lead to a more co-ordinated and efficient heart contraction as well as a genuine increase in contractile force; although herbalists have used foxglove for centuries for this effect, especially in cases of dropsy (i.e., the oedema that follows right heart failure), in modern times the remedy lily-of-the valley is preferred as providing a more gentle action and lowered neurotoxicity, due to the particular balance of cardioactive glycosides in the whole plant. Other plants that contain cardioactive glycosides include broom, squills and figwort, but it is not clear how this action plays a part in that of the whole plant. On a broader level, there are other remedies with actions on the heart not due to cardioactive glycosides: these are often of a more gentle tonifying action and the term 'cardiotonic' has been used for them; they include hawthorn, motherwort, rosemary, ephedra, and possibly (though there are doubts as to its exact action and safety) mistletoe.

Carduus benedictus, blessed thistle.

Carduus marianus, milk thistle.

---

carminative, a term used to denote a remedy that eases flatulence and colic in the gut; generally a property of **volatile oils** of a certain type, though conceivably resulting from the action of other plant constituents; the principle action seems to be a soothing, settling effect on the gut wall. Notable carminative plants include aniseed, cardamom, cinnamon, dill, fennel, ginger, cassia, lovage, parsley, pennyroyal, peppermint, sassafras, thyme, wintergreen, asafoetida, catmint, celery, galanga, hyssop, jambul, motherwort, sweet flag, wood sage.

---

carrot, wild, Queen Anne's lace, *Daucus carota* L. Fam: Umbelliferae.
An erect biennial up to 1 metre high with narrow divided and pinnatifid leaves and large crowded umbels, often concave and globular after flowering; fruits ovoid and covered with prickles on their ribs, the 4

secondary ribs more prominent than the 3 primaries; the aroma and taste is very like the cultivated plant.

Habitat: indigenous to maritime chalky soils of southern Europe but has spread widely, partly through reversion from cultivated plants; prefers sea coasts but found almost anywhere.

Constituents: volatile oil, alkaloid (daucine).

Actions: diuretic and having other effects on the urinary system.

Applications: to urinary calculi and infections; oedema.

Dosage: 1-4 grams of dried herb three times per day.

Carum carvi, caraway.

Carum petroselinum, parsley.

---

cascara sagrada, *Rhamnus purshiana* D.C. Fam: Rhamnaceae.

The bark of shrubby deciduous tree between 5 and 8 metres high, with alternate dark-green, irregularly-toothed or entire, elliptical or oblong leaves and small greenish flowers growing in umbels; the reddish bark when dried is found as quilled or curved pieces, smooth on the outside, often with lichen and moss fragments still attached, with yellow-to-black inner surface; the taste is bitter and persistent.

Habitat: mountainous areas of north-west North America.

Constituents: anthraquinone glycosides (including emodin, chrysophanic acid, aloe-emodin, cascarosides A, B, C and D); tannin; volatile oil (rhamnol).

Actions: stimulating laxative, with a gentler action than others in its class.

Applications: atonic constipation.

Dosage: 1-3 grams of well-dried bark equivalent before retiring.

---

cassia bark, Chinese cinnamon, *Cinnamomum cassia* Blume. Fam: Lauraceae.

The bark of an evergreen tree with large flame-coloured leaves and delicate blossom; the bark is obtained in quills of a dull yellow-brown colour with scars on the outer surface and with a fragrant odour reminiscent of cinnamon, but with a stronger taste.

Habitat: indigenous to China and South-East Asia

Constituents: volatile oil (including cinnamaldehyde), tannin.

Actions: warming and soothing; carminative; antispasmodic.

Applications: for the effects of cold, especially when associated with loss of appetite, diarrhoea, weakness; for flatulence and griping pains in the abdomen.

Dosage: 0.5-1 gram dried bark equivalent three times per day.

Cassia spp,   senna.

Castanea sativa et spp,   chestnut, sweet.

---

catarrh, an excessive mucous secretion from the respiratory mucosa; a term also used in naturopathy to denote a toxic congestive condition of other mucosal tissues. Catarrh of the respiratory system can occur in the lower system (i.e., below the larynx) and is relieved by the use of **expectorants** (*see also* **bronchitis** and **cough**): upper respiratory catarrh may be relieved with the use of such remedies as ground ivy, eyebright, ribwort, goldenrod, elderflowers and hyssop, as well as steam inhalations to which are added chamomile flowers, and small levels of volatile oils like cinnamon, eucalyptus and pine. Peppermint oils should be used only for very severe congestion, and never for too long. Whereas these remedies will relieve catarrh, full treatment of the condition will depend on background factors: there are two approaches, each appropriate to one of two quite distinct types of catarrh. The first, the more common, was traditionally termed 'cold', in modern times 'vagotonic': it is found in those of sluggish metabolism who like stodgy, sweet food and dairy products, feel cold easily and like warmth; the catarrh tends to be watery and copious, the mucous membranes pale and puffy; the common **cold** is a frequent complication, and it is often associated with **bronchitis** as well. Background treatment of such conditions will emphasize **circulatory stimulants** (the 'warming' remedies). The second form of catarrh, the 'hot' type or 'sympatheticotonic' type is linked with an active constitution and high metabolic rate, possibly a nervous or 'hyped-up' personality; the catarrh is thicker and more scanty and the affected mucous membranes are more inflamed. Background treatment may concentrate on giving **bitters, relaxants,** or in extreme cases, **sedatives** (the 'cooling' remedies). In all cases of catarrh, exposure to smoke and air-borne irritants must be minimized, alcohol consumption cut well back, and sweets, starchy foods and milk products eliminated. Fruit is cleansing and beneficial for the mucous membranes, and, especially when taken warmed, fruit juice provides quick relief.

---

catechu, black,   Cutch, *Acacia catechu* Willd. Fam: Legiminosae.
The dried extract obtained from the heartwood of a tree of the acacia family; it is sold in black cakes that break showing a dark-brown, glossy porous surface.
Habitat: Burma, Bangladesh and eastern India.
Constituents: high levels of tannins (mainly catechutannic acid), flavonoids, red pigment.
Actions: strongly astringent.
Applications: to diarrhoea and gut infections and irritations; locally, as a douche for vaginal and cervical affections, and as a mouthwash and gargle for gum, mouth and throat infections and inflammations.
Dosage: 0.3-2 grams of dried extract equivalent three times per day.

Note: pale catechu (*Uncaria gambier* Roxb.) may be used in the same way: it is however slightly less astringent.

---

cathartic,   a term denoting a remedy that produces a positive evacuation from the bowels; *see* **laxative.**

---

catmint,   Catnep, Catnip, *Nepeta cataria* L. Fam: Labiatae
An erect, shrubby herb up to 100cm in height with whitish-green serrated ovate leaves with hairy undersides; the flowers are white to pale blue, dotted with crimson, arranged in small tight whorls with toothed hairy sepals; the odour is characteristically mint-like and much appreciated by cats
Habitat: banks, waysides and waste places on calcareous soils throughout all northern temperate regions.
Constituents: volatile oil, bitter principle, tannins.
Actions: gentle stimulant of the circulation though in fever actually acting to reduce body temperature (*see* **fever remedies**); relieving congestions in the upper respiratory pathways; relaxant and carminative; digestive stimulant; astringent.
Applications: to colds, upper respiratory affections and fevers, particularly where there is a feeling of congestion in the airways, sinuses or middle ear; nervous dyspepsia and a wide range of digestive upsets.
Dosage: 1-4 grams of the dried herb equivalent three times per day.

Caulophyllum thalictroides,   blue cohosh.

---

cayenne, Chillies, Red pepper, Bird pepper, *Capsicum minimum* Roxb., *C. frutescens* L. Fam: Solanaceae.

The familiar red and hot spice, available in small pods or as powder.

Habitat: a native of tropical America and now cultivated in Africa as well.

Constituents: alkaloid (capsaicin), carotene pigment (capsanthine), flavonoids, ascorbic acid, volatile oil.

Actions: a strong circulatory stimulant, appearing to reinforce the action of certain prostaglandins so as to markedly increase the blood flow through all tissues of the body and to increase the subjective feeling of heat; thus a strong diaphoretic; also stimulates gastric secretions and acts as a carminative; antiseptic; counter-irritant.

Applications: to supporting the treatment of any condition marked by reduced circulation and/or a feeling of cold, acting to 'flush out' diseased tissues and helping to reverse pathological deteriorations; to colic and flatulent dyspepsia, and digestive debility in general; locally as a counter-irritant for joint inflammations, neuralgia. A central remedy in the North American tradition, *see* **physiomedicalism.**

Dosage: 30-120mg dried fruits equivalent three times a day.

Caution: not to be used in cases of gastric hyperacidity or on mucous membranes.

celandine, greater, Garden celandine, *Chelidonium majus* L. Fam: Papaveraceae.

The leaves of a perennial plant related to the poppies with erect slender branching stems up to 60cm high; the thin pale-green smooth leaves are pinnate with toothed or lobed segments and with stalks often dilated into false stipules; small yellow are in groups of 3-6 in loose umbels giving way to smooth cylindrical seed pods; these and the stems produce a yellow foetid sap when cut.

Habitat: on waysides and waste places, and near habitation, in Britain, Europe, Asia and north-eastern North America.

Constituents: alkaloids (including chelidonine, chelerythrin, protopine, sanguinarine); bitter principle; volatile oil.

Actions: cholagogue and bitter; antispasmodic; diuretic; laxative.

Applications: to gallstones and gall-bladder and biliary diseases; as a constituent of prescriptions designed to clear the liver and bowel.

Dosage: 1-2 grams of dried herb three times per day.

Caution: although generally safe in therapeutic doses this plant is best avoided by untrained persons (under the terms of the Medicines Act 1968 its sale is restricted to medical herbalists).

celery, Smallage, *Apium graveolens* L. Fam: Umbelliferae.
The seed of a biennial slender plant up to 60cm in height, with 3-5 segmented pinnate leaves, each segment with three lobes; the umbels are small and nearly sessile without many bracts, the flower petals are small, white and with a small inflected point; the fruits (or seeds) are very small and slightly compressed laterally; their odour is very distinctive.

Habitat: grows wild in maritime districts in northern warm or temperate zones and inland as a naturalized escape from cultivation.

Constituents: volatile oil (including apiol), bergapten, flavonoids (including apiin), fixed oil.

Actions: increases the elimination of uric acid, and possibly other acids through the kidneys; urinary antiseptic; digestive tonic and carminative; uterine stimulant; galactogogue.

Applications: to arthritic conditions associated with acidic accumulations and/or urinary infections or calculi; notably for gout; to stimulate milk flow.

Dosage: 1-3 grams of dried fruit (seed) equivalent three times per day.

Caution: to be avoided in pregnancy.

Note: seed sold for horticultural use is usually dressed with fungicide: do not use.

Centaurium erythraea, centaury.

---

centaury, *Centaurium erythraea* Rafin., *Erythraea centaurium* L. Fam: Gentianaceae.

A small erect annual or biennial herb from 2 to 30cm high, branching considerably at the top and arising out of a tuft of small broad ovate leaves; numerous pink or red flowers arise in a terminal cyme or panicle; the taste is bitter; there are several subspecies recognized.

Habitat: dry shady banks, waysides and pastures over Britain, Europe and Asia.

Constituents: bitter glycosides (including gentiopicrine and erythrocentaurin), alkaloid (gentianine), volatile oil, resin, flavonoids.

Actions: bitter and hepatic.

Applications: to debilated digestion, especially in children; to help digestion and reduce body temperature in fevers.

Dosage: 1-4 grams of dried herb equivalent three times per day.

Centella asiatica, gotu kola.

Cephaelis ipecacuanha et spp, ipecacuanha.

---

cervical problems, causing discharge, or pain on deep penetration; most often 'erosion' or infection, occasionally carcinoma; must therefore be checked with a 'Pap' smear. Treatment of erosion or infection in herbal terms is generally by douche (*see* **vaginal problems**).

Cetraria islandica, Iceland moss.

Chamaelirium luteum et spp, helonias root.

Chamaemelum nobile, Chamomile, Roman.

---

chamomile, Roman, True or perennial chamomile, *Anthemis nobilis* L., *Chamaemelum nobile* L. Fam: Compositae.

The flowerheads of a perennial, rather short and stocky plant, sometimes actually creeping, with pinnate leaves, and typical yellow and white flowers on terminal peduncles. The raised yellow receptacle is solid throughout. The odour is strong and characteristic.

Details of this remedy are similar to those for wild chamomile (*see below*). Although this has traditionally been the herbalist's favourite, to the point of there being a specially cultivated double-flowered variety that is most highly regarded, in practice there is little to distinguish between the actions of this flower and the wild chamomile.

---

chamomile, wild, German chamomile, *Matricaria recutita (M. chamomilla)* L. Fam: Compositae.

The flowerheads of an annual rather wispy plant up to 60cm in height, with slender bi- and tripinnate leaves; the yellow raised receptacle is hollow, and surrounded by white ligulate florets; the odour is strong and characteristic.

Habitat: found in fields and open ground throughout the temperate regions of the northern hemisphere.

Constituents: volatile oil (including the azulenes, bisabolol, farnesine and other sesquiterpenes); sesquiterpene lactones; cyanogenic glycosides; acetylenic salicylate derivatives; valerianic acid; flavonoids; tannins.

Action: the flowers are notable for their relaxant properties, calming restlessness, and tensions, particularly as they affect the viscera such as the digestive tract; they also have the properties of their **bitterness** and thus stimulate digestive secretions; they are anti-inflammatory, reducing especially the results of allergic responses; they reduce the intensity of many gynaecological problems, notably dysmenorrhoea; they share many of the constituents and **peripheral vasodilatory** properties of **yarrow** and are thus applicable to fever management.

Application: to all states of tension and the visceral symptoms that can arise therefrom, such as nervous dyspepsia and nervous bowel, tension headaches, and sleeplessness; especially useful for all **children's** conditions, calming without depressing; to calming period pains and menopausal tensions; to **fever management**; as an **inhalation** for catarrhal and allergic conditions of the airways; for locally healing applications and poultices.

Dosage: 1-4 grams dried flowers equivalent three times or more per day.

Chelidonium majus, celandine, greater.

Chelone glabra, balmony.

---

chestnut, horse, *Aesculus hippocastanum* L. Fam: Hippocastanaceae.
The fruit of a large erect tree with spreading branches producing in autumn large sticky leaf buds that open in spring into large palmate leaves with five or seven leaflets, all with finely toothed margins; the flowers are in prominent upright spikes, white or pink, with a strong fragrance; the fruit is a large shiny brown nut, enclosed in a large spiny seed-capsule.

Habitat: indigenous to Western Asia, spreading to Europe and now widely cultivated around the world as an ornamental tree.

Constituents: triterpenoid saponins (including aescine), flavonoids (including aesculetin), tannin, coumarin glycoside (aesculoside).

Actions: astringent and antihaemorrhagic; tonic to venous walls; diuretic; anti-inflammatory.

Applications: to varicosed veins and haemorrhoids, both locally and systemically; to phlebitis; to managing enteric infections, diarrhoea and fevers arising therefrom; to prostatic enlargement.

Dosage: 0.2-1 gram of dried fruits equivalent three times per day.

---

chestnut, sweet, Spanish chestnut, European chestnut, *Castanea sativa* Mill., *C. vulgaris* Lam. Fam: Fagaceae.

The leaves of a very large, stately tree with male and female catkins producing 2-3 chestnuts enclosed in a spiny casket; the leaves are large, narrow and glossy, pointed at both ends, with sharp teeth on the margins, and prominent veins.

Habitat: throughout south-west and southern Europe and south-west Asia; common in England.

Constituents: tannins, flavonoids, resin, pectin.

Actions: relaxing expectorant; astringent; anti-inflammatory.

Applications: to paroxysmal, irritating, nervous and non-productive coughs; to myalgias, fibrositis and 'muscular rheumatism'; to managing diarrhoea and fevers of enteric or pulmonary origin.

Dosage: 1-4 grams of dried leaves equivalent three times per day.

---

chicken pox, or varicella, a generally mild and very common infective disease of children, produced by the body's reaction to the same virus that produces **shingles** in adults; the condition is recognized by rashes, turning into crops of spots quickly becoming blistered, pustular and finally scabbed, mostly on scalp, in mouth and on trunk, and very irritating; accompanying fever is relatively low grade; recovery is generally within a fortnight; treatment is thus conservative (*see* **fever management**), but extra **relaxant** measures and local applications (*see* **pruritus**) may be necessary to avoid excessive scratching.

---

chickweed, Starweed, *Stellaria media* (L) Vill. Fam: Caryophyllaceae.

A soft, sappy branched annual, smooth except for a line of hairs down the stem, with small ovate and pointed leaves, the lower stalked and heart-shaped, the upper sessile and narrower; small white flowers occur on rather long stalks; the taste is mucilaginous.

Habitat: cultivated and waste ground, waysides and streambanks throughout all temperate regions of the world.

Constituents: mucilage, anti-inflammatory saponins.

Actions: soothing and astringent.

Applications: as an external application to soothe inflamed, erupted and especially itchy skin conditions.

---

chilblains, essentially a mild form of frostbite, a spasm of the small blood vessels to the periphery in reaction to lowering of the outside temperature; dull-red, itchy swellings at the extremities, occasionally breaking; external measures which reduce the impact of changes in temperature are useful (e.g., woollen socks and gloves, moderate even heating); herbal treatment emphasizes the use of **peripheral vasodilators** and **circulatory stimulants**; it can be very effective.

children's remedies, there are many herbs particularly appropriate to children's conditions, combining gentleness of action and a supportive restorative core with genuine effectiveness. Many herbs, however, are ruled out on the grounds of taste and this category often includes herbs that are rather too dynamic for ready use in children. The dosage of the remedy will obviously be lower (a quarter adult dose up to the age of two years, rising through a third to half adult dose around the age of eight to ten years; then quickly rising to an adult regime soon after puberty); however, for the following recommended herbs relatively larger doses are possible without harm. For most complaints, relaxing remedies like chamomile, limeflowers, lemon balm and peppermint are almost central to treatment; for coughs, hyssop, elderflowers and licorice are recommended; for fever, yarrow, elderflower and catmint are excellent regulators (*see* **fever management**); digestive upsets will respond to chamomile, peppermint, cinnamon, fennel or dill; catarrhal conditions to ground ivy, ribwort and elderflower; urinary problems to couch grass or corn silk; nervous exhaustion to oats, vervain, angelica or chamomile; gentle 'warming' or circulatory stimulation is possible with cinnamon, cardamom, angelica or even fresh ginger; constipation must *never* be treated with stimulating laxatives, and chamomile, dill, fennel and other **relaxant** measures are necessary instead (*see* **constipation**).

Chimaphila umbellata, pipisissewa.

chiretta, Indian gentian, Indian balmony, *Swertia chirata* Buch-Ham. Fam: Gentianaceae.
   An annual plant about 1 metre in height with narrow pointed, smooth opposite leaves, and numerous yellow flowers; the taste is extremely bitter.
   Habitat: northern India and Nepal.
   Constituents: bitter principles (chiratin, ophelic acid); xanthones (no tannins).

Actions: strong digestive and hepatic stimulant.

Applications: debility and cachexic conditions marked by lowered appetite and digestive performance; gall-bladder disease; formerly used for malaria.

Dosage: 0.3-2 grams of dried herb three times a day.

---

cholagogue,   a remedy that stimulates the flow of bile from the liver; generally a property of the **bitters,** but produced by other plant constituents as well; cholagogues are used to improve the cleansing of the liver and to aid it in removing material from the body as excretion in the bile (to this end they are often combined with **laxatives,** and formerly **emetics**); they thus make up an important part of an **eliminative** regime, and of the treatment of **liver disease,** and wider liver dysfunction. Notable cholagogues include celandine, barberry, chiretta, artichoke, birch, blue flag, golden seal, rosemary, sage, wild indigo, butternut, boldo, boneset, curled dock, balmony and dandelion. *See also* **hepatics.**

Chondrus crispus,   Irish moss.

Chrysanthemum partenium,   feverfew.

Chrysanthemum vulgare,   tansy.

Cimicifuga racemosa,   black cohosh.

---

cinchona,   Peruvian bark, Jesuit's bark, Red bark, *Cinchona succirubra* Pav., *C. officinalis* L., *C. ledgeriana* Moens., *C. calisaya* Wedd. Fam: Rubiaceae.

The bark of several species and hybrids of evergreen tree obtained as quills or curved pieces with outer fissured and roughened grey surface often bearing lichens and mosses, with an inner surface of a deep reddish-brown; the taste is bitter and astringent.

Habitat: hot regions in tropical South America, but hybrids are cultivated in India, Sri Lanka, and South-East Asia.

Constituents: alkaloids (including quinine, quinidine, cinchonine, hydroquinine); bitter glycoside (quinovin); quinic acid; tannins; cinchona red.

Actions: bitter digestive and hepatic stimulant; antiprotozoal; reducing irritability in striated muscle; stimulant to the gravid uterus; diaphoretic and febrifuge.

Applications: to malaria; to many hepatic conditions giving rise to enlarged spleen; to loss of appetite and other debilitated conditions of digestion; for night cramps and cardiac arrythmias; for any severe fever when body temperature rises too high; for drunkenness.

Dosage: 0.1-0.25 gram of dried bark equivalent three times per day. Maximum legal dose is 0.25 gram.

Caution: the remedy must not be used in pregnancy, or in any case for too long (it is likely to depress the reticuloendothelial defence system in excess); it is incompatible with remedies containing salicylates. In the U.K. it may only be sold to practitioners.

Cinchona spp, cinchona.

Cinnamomum cassia, cassia bark.

Cinnamomum zeylanicum, cinnamon.

---

cinnamon, *Cinnamomum zeylanicum* Blume. Fam: Lauraceae.
The inner bark of a tree reaching 10 metres in height with leathery leaves and panicles of small white flowers; it is bought as single or double quills of pink-to-yellow-brown colour with outer surface marked by ridges and scars; the taste and aroma are fragrant and characteristic.

Habitat: Sri Lanka, but cultivated in South-East Asia.

Constituents: volatile oil (including cinnamic aldehyde, eugenol and phellandrene); condensed tannins.

Actions: carminative; gentle warming digestive tonic; antispasmodic.

Applications: flatulent dyspepsia; digestive atony associated with cold and debilitated conditions; intestinal colic and bowel looseness.

Dosage: 0.3-1 gram of dried bark equivalent three times per day.

---

circulatory stimulants, plants whose action on the body involves the increase of blood flow through the tissues of the body; the important constituents in such plants seem to include certain **volatile oils, alkaloids,** and **mustard oil glycosides;** the key action has occasionally been shown to involve prostaglandin and kinin stimulation. The result of circulatory stimulation is a feeling of warmth and an actual raising of temperature in the tissues: the implications can both be speculated on and justified; the increased blood flow brings increased oxygen and nourishment to the tissues (and pathological deterioration always commences with a severe reduction in oxygen to the diseased tissue); it brings an increased input of defensive white blood cells (with evidence of an increased activity on their part as well); and it flushes out cell metabolites and waste products more efficiently. Such activity helps to account for the traditional claims that circulatory stimulants quite simply support vitality in the tissues and reduce the impact of toxicity. These claims refer to the ancient association of life (and thus health) with heat and fire, the latter images best conveying the positive, transforming, transcending, warming and powerful qualities of the life force (and the mundane observation that, on death, the body cools); remedies that were 'hot' were seen as increasing the body's heat, and quite literally its vitality (*see* **physiomedicalism** and **fever managements**); they were particularly applied when the disease was seen as being 'cold' in nature, that is when the patient feels the cold easily, when the condition is relieved by the application of heat, when the complexion is pale, the demeanour quiet and withdrawn, the tongue wet, pale and with a white coating, and he produces copious catarrh and dilute urine. In practice this means that they are often applied in cases of the common cold and associated conditions, and in many cases of fever and inflammation (where their action reduces the need for painful histamine-mediated inflammatory response, *see* **inflammation**), but their use can be considered in almost any case where the criteria fit: such is the pivotal nature of circulatory stimulation in improving normal tissue health that it is very often possible *to bring about health with this measure alone*. Remedies of this group (classified as 'hot in the second and third degrees' in the Galenic classification) include all the hot spices such as cayenne, horseradish, the mustards, ginger, galanga and, to a lesser extent, raw garlic, cinnamon, angelica root, cardamom, bayberry, blood root, cassia, echinacea, fennel, kava-kava, lovage, figwort, Siberian ginseng, lavender, rosemary, elecampane, blue flag, condurango, queen's delight, betony, white horehound, nettle, sarsaparilla, sassafras, wild indigo, Oregon grape and rue. The use of any of these remedies should be considered in this context, and perhaps limited if the condition is already too 'hot' (as defined in the discussion of **bitters** and notably in those very young and excitable in disposition). *See also* **peripheral vasodilators**.

---

cleavers,   Clivers, Goosegrass, Hedge-burs, Sticky-willie, Cleaverwort,

Galium aparine L. Fam: Rubiaceae.

A straggling annual, scrambling through bushes and hedges, clinging to them, and to anyone brushing them, by tiny curved prickles on the angles of the stems and the veins and edges of the 2-3cm thin lanceolate leaves; these occur in whorls of 6-8 encircling the stem; the small greenish-white flowers are borne in peduncles from the axils of each whorl; the fruits are round, forming small burs of 4-6mm covered with hooked bristles.

Habitat: a common hedgerow plant throughout Britain, Europe, Canada, the eastern half of the U.S.A. and the Pacific coast of that continent.

Constituents: coumarins, asperuloside, red dye (including galiosin), tannins, citric acid.

Actions: diuretic and lymphatic alterative.

Applications: an effective remedy for skin eruptions, lymphadenopathy, and other toxic conditions, especially where associated with tissue oedema and water retention; for urinary infections, calculi, colic and strangury.

Dosage: 2-8 grams of dried herb equivalent three times per day.

Cnicus benedictus,   blessed thistle.

Cochlearia armoracia,   horseradish.

---

cola,   *see* **kola.**

Cola vera et spp,   kola.

---

cold, common,   the result of invasion of the upper respiratory mucous membranes by certain types of virus. These viruses constantly circulate in the atmosphere in enclosed and especially public spaces, so everyone is frequently in contact with them. When a cold actually occurs, therefore, it is because the sufferer has allowed the virus access: we do not 'catch colds' by accident. The opposite also holds: the much-sought-after 'cure for the common cold' is to be found within everyone who does not have a cold — it is normal vital resistance to the viral intrusion. Thus colds are seen by herbalists as weaknesses in mucosal defences. They are treated initially as for **catarrh** with particular emphasis on the 'cold' or 'vagotonic' type. In practice a cold may be held at bay by frequent sipping of a cup of hot water with cinnamon and fresh ginger (a teaspoon of each per cup) with fresh lemon juice.

'cold' remedies,   *see* **bitters, relaxants** and **sedatives.**

---

cold sores,   *see* **herpes.**

---

colic,   sharp bouts of cramping pain in the abdomen, most often caused by functional spasm of the gut (*see* **flatulence, nervous bowel**), but possibly indicates more serious conditions such as gut infections, adhesions, **appendicitis,** strangulated hernia, lead poisoning, cancer, so should be checked if persistent or puzzling; colicky pains also accompany gallstones (*see* **gall-bladder disease**), **urinary stones,** painful **menstruation,** or complications of pregnancy.

---

colitis, mucous,   *see* **nervous bowel.**

---

colitis, ulcerative,   an intermittent or chronic inflammation of the large bowel with ulceration. Marked by diarrhoea with the passage of blood and mucus, pain and often fever (all the symptoms of **dysentery**). An example of an **auto-immune** disorder and thus of great complexity. Severe phases of the disease will sometimes require conventional drug treatment and the condition will always require expert attention. Emphasis will be placed on looking for deep underlying causes, often far away from the bowel itself, reducing potential food allergens (*see* **food allergies**) especially gluten and milk, cutting out rough or 'pippy' roughage like seeds and nuts, and treating with herbal remedies such as **astringents** or **mucilages.**

Collinsonia canadensis,   stone root.

---

colombo,   *see* **calumba.**

---

coltsfoot,   Coughwort, Horsehoof, *Tussilago farfara* L. Fam: Compositae.

The flowers and leaves of a prolific herb with creeping rootstock, giving rise to the characteristic hairy flowering stem in mid-winter; each produces a single yellow flower 15-35mm in diameter, converting to a white downy sphere at the same time as the large leaves appear.

Habitat: a common invasive weed, found especially on heavy clay soils throughout Britain, Europe, North Africa and Asia and sporadically in North America; it is also found wild in damp areas, river banks and ditches.

Constituents: mucilage, tannins (little in flowers), bitter principle, hormonal substances, zinc.

Actions: relaxing **expectorant** particularly effective in reducing non-productive coughs, and soothing dry and irritable airways; locally an excellent healing and soothing remedy.

Applications: to 'hot, dry cough and for wheezings and shortness of breath' (Parkinson) a notable standby for children's coughs and other cases where there is a nervous and spasmodic element to the symptom; in all such cases will make the cough more productive.

Dosage: 0.6-2 grams of the dried flowers equivalent three times a day; the leaves are less effective and may be taken up to doses of 4 grams.

---

comfrey, Knitbone, Boneset, Blackwort, Bruisewort, *Symphytum officinale* L. Fam: Boraginaceae.

The root and leaves of a vigorous plant with broadly lanceolate leaves up to 30cm long arising as a rosette from the ground, with rough texture and covered with short stiff hairs; the rosette supports a tall flowering stem up to 1.5 metres in height, covered with sessile leaves and bearing forked stalks supporting one-sided racemes of pedicillate bell-shaped mauve or white flowers curving downwards; the root is thick, quite short and very branched, black on the outside with a white interior and extremely mucilaginous. The Russian comfrey (*S. peregrinum*), widely grown for its horticultural benefits can also be used.

Habitat: on moist banks, field borders, ditches and watersides throughout Britain, Europe, western Asia and the U.S.A.

Constituents: mucilage and gum, allantoin, tannins, resin, pyrrolizidine alkaloids.

Actions: effective stimulant to fibroblast, chondroblast and osteoblast activity; soothing and astringent; relaxing expectorant.

Applications: an impressive local healing agent for wounds, slow-healing ulcers, internal wounds, strains and bone fractures (due variously to mixture of binding mucilage-tannin mixture, and the highly diffusable stimulant of connective tissue, bone and cartilage — allantoin); taken internally for ulceration and erosion of the gut wall; for bronchitic conditions.

Dosage: 1-4 grams of dried root or leaf equivalent three times per day.

Caution: the presence of hepatotoxic pyrrolizidine alkaloids has raised doubts over the safety of this remedy; such doubts are likely to be ill-founded, especially for the leaves, but to be safe it is better that excessive internal consumption be avoided.

---

comminution, the grinding of herbal material to convenient size, either powder or large pieces; the pestle and mortar were the traditional implements but modern machinery is most often used today.

Commiphora molmol, myrrh.

---

condurango, Eagle vine, *Marsdenia condurango* Rchb. Fam: Asclepiadaceae.

The bark of a tall robust vine available commercially as curved and quilled pieces with outer surface light grey to brown, rough and warty, and inner surface paler and longitudinally striated; with a slightly aromatic odour and bitter taste.

Habitat: Ecuador and Peru.

Constituents: glycosides ('condurangin'), tannin, resin.

Actions: digestive stimulant; alterative; circulatory stimulant.

Applications: to gastric inflammations and irritation, particularly where associated with diminished appetite and digestive performance or dietary abuse; to anorexia nervosa.

Dosage: 0.5-3 grams of dried bark equivalent three times per day.

---

conjunctivitis, *see* **eye problems.**

---

constipation, sluggish emptying of the bowels, usually with dry and hard stools. Two distinct varieties: the more common flaccid or atonic condition, arising from low-fibre diets, lack of exercise and long-term neglect of the urge to defaecation; and the tense, nervous or spastic condition, where tension is transferred onto the bowel muscle, interfering with free natural movement therein. This latter condition is marked by being found more in young people or those of nervous constitution, worsening in periods of stress, often alternating with periods of looseness (*see* **nervous bowel**), and occasionally leading to the production of small nut-like stools and/or mucus. The two problems *must be treated differently.* Atonic constipation may be treated in the short term with **anthraquinone laxatives;** in the long term, often over a period of many months, normal bowel function can be restored with a high-fibre diet, exercise or massage, and a teaspoonful twice daily of a powdered mixture of 4 parts of psyllium seed, 2 parts chamomile flowers and 1 part of alder buckthorn bark. Tense constipation *must not* be treated with anthraquinone laxatives as this will only increase underlying tension. Instead **visceral relaxants** should be prescribed, and sometimes it is worth dropping bran from the diet and replacing it by softer sources of roughage. Constipation is seen by the herbalist as a significant source of reabsorbed toxic material and is thus always accorded high priority in any treatment.

convalescence, a term now little used in modern medicine, but still most applicable to the approach of the herbalist. Briefly, it is assumed that after any undue stress on the vital reserves of the body a period of recovery will be needed wherein any depletion can be corrected. In cases of severe illness or trauma this period may be many months, whilst in a non-serious **fever** it may only be a day or two. During convalescence adequate rest is essential, with a freedom from usual daily strains (a holiday is ideal); food should be moderate, healthy and sustaining, there should be plenty of fresh air, adequate fluid intake, but little or no caffeine, alcohol, nicotine or other stimulants. Herbs are most useful, and a choice is made from the most restorative and tonic, notably angelica root, oatstraw, vervain, St John's wort, rosemary, yarrow, damiana and **bitters,** or heating remedies like cayenne or ginger if appropriate.

Convallaria majalis, Lily-of-the-valley.

convulsions, or fits, can occur in a wide variety of situations; in children they may herald or accompany **fevers** or almost any other internal problem; in the adult such a reaction is likely to manifest as rigors rather than full convulsions: full adult convulsions may signal **epilepsy** or brain injury or disease (e.g., meningitis or encephalitis), tetanus, kidney failure, alcoholism, or may be the result of intense emotional or psychological trauma. Obviously, most such cases are too serious to be treated lightly, but it may be helpful as part of a wider treatment to use such remedies as cramp bark, scullcap, passion flower or valerian to reduce the intensity of the convulsions.

corn silk, *Zea mays* L. Fam: Graminaceae.

The stigmas and styles obtained from the corn or maize plant before the corn is ripe; when fresh they are like silken threads of a light green or yellow-brown colour, but dry to fine dark crinkled hairs; there is little taste or odour.

Habitat: indigenous to central America, but widely cultivated elsewhere.

Constituents: saponins, volatile alkaloid, sterols, allantoin, tannins, resin.

Actions: diuretic with soothing influence on the urinary mucosa.

Applications: to urinary infections and calculi.

Dosage: 2-8 grams of dried styles and stigmas equivalent three times per day.

---

coronary disease, *see* **heart problems.**

---

cotton root, *Gossypium herbaceum* L. *et spp* Fam: Malvaceae.

The bark of the root of a biennial or perennial plant up to 2 metres in height with hairy leaves divided into narrow lobes and yellow flowers with a central purple spot giving rise to the seed capsule that reveals a tuft of cotton when open; the root bark is very light coloured and occurs in often very long thin fibrous strips, with slight characteristic odour when fresh and a sweet and acrid taste.

Habitat: indigenous to India but various species are grown throughout Asia, southern Europe and the U.S.A.

Constituents: phenolic glycoside (gossypol), tannins, resin (with phenols), salicylates

Actions: uterine stimulant; depressing testicular production.

Applications: to suppressed menstruation and congestive dysmenorrhoea; formerly used to encourage labour contractions but not now recommended for this purpose; shown to reduce markedly the sperm count in men taking it but full safety and efficacy as a male contraceptive not established.

Dosage: 1-4 grams of dried root bark equivalent three times per day.

Caution: a potent abortifacient so not to be used during pregnancy.

---

couch grass, Twitch, Scutch, Witchgrass, Quick grass, *Agropyron repens* Beav., *Triticum repens* L. Fam: Graminaceae.

The extensive rhizomes of this pervasive perennial grass; with hollow stems except at the nodes and leaves completely ensheathing the stem: at the top of each sheath where it joins with the leaf blade is a tiny stiff appendage known as a ligule, about 1mm in length. The rhizome is available as short yellow-brown hard pieces with longitudinal furrows.

Habitat: on cultivated land in temperate climates almost everywhere.

Constituents: mannitol, large quantities of silica, mucilage, gum, vanillin, saponin, antibiotic substance (agropyrene), iron and other minerals (all such plants that 'rob' the land of its minerals have this advantage).

Actions: a soothing diuretic, calming pain and spasm in the urinary tract.

Applications: an excellent basic remedy for the control of the symptoms of urinary diseases, from infections to the results of calculi and even prostatic disease; its symptomatic effect seems to be augmented by a genuine healing action on the urinary mucosa; particularly effective for children's conditions and helping to manage examples of tension in the urinary system, e.g., enuresis and nervous incontinence.

Dosage: 1-4 grams of dried rhizome equivalent three or more times per day.

---

cough, a sign of irritation or blockage of the bronchial tubes and of the body's attempts to expel same. Rather than simply seeking to suppress the cough with 'anti-tussive' medicines, the herbalist seeks to help the eliminative process by helping the cough in its job; thus using, depending on the type of cough, either stimulating or relaxing **expectorants.** In cases where the cough is clearly counter-productive (as in nervous coughing or when there is an immovable irritant such as an injury or cancer) then anti-tussive remedies may be tried: wild cherry bark, anise, and such sedatives as wild lettuce.

---

cowslip, Paigle, *Primula veris* L. *Primula officinalis* (L) Hill. Fam: Primulaceae.

The dried flowers of a perennial herb, one of three races of *Primula veris* (with the primrose and true oxlip), with a rosette of oblong toothed leaves, narrowing abruptly below the middle; the flowerstalks rise above the leaves bearing an umbel of cup-shaped yellow flowers.

Habitat: in grassland in temperate regions of Britain, Europe and Asia.

Constituents: saponins (including primulic acid), glycosides (including primulaveroside and primveroside, containing salicylates), essential oil ('primula camphor') flavonoids.

Actions: stimulating expectorant; antispasmodic; sedative.

Applications: to nervous excitation and insomnia; to congestive

bronchial conditions, such as chronic bronchitis and whooping cough.
Dosage: 0.5-2 grams of dried flowers equivalent three times per day.

---

cramp bark, Guelder rose, European cranberry, *Viburnum opulus* L.
Fam: Caprifoliaceae.

The stem bark of a shrub or small tree, being the wild form of a common garden cultivar; the large, broad 3-5 pointed shiny leaves are on slender leafstalks, the small white flowers borne in dense cymes giving way to black or red globular drupes. The bark is available in quills or powder, of a pale reddish-brown colour.

Habitat: in hedgerows and woods over Europe and Russian Asia, and freely naturalized in North America.

Constituents: a bitter (viburnin), valerianic acid, salicosides, tannin and a resin.

Action: a smooth and skeletal muscle relaxant, possibly acting on innervation as well as through a local effect.

Applications: valuable as a specific remedy for visceral tensions, where visceral smooth muscle is manifesting states of increased activity; such conditions include colicky conditions of the gut, biliary apparatus and urinary system, some cases of migraine and other conditions of vasospasm (such as drastic interference in peripheral circulation, to the hands and feet), asthmatic conditions, **dysphagia, dysmenorrhoea,** nervous **dyspepsia** and **nervous bowel** problems. It may also be used to help quieten convulsive states in children. Locally, it makes an excellent application for states of skeletal muscle tension or cramp.

Dosage: 1-4 grams of the dried bark equivalent three times a day.

---

cranesbill, American, Wild geranium, Alumroot, Storksbill, Spotted cranesbill, *Geranium maculatum* L. Fam: Geraniaceae.

The rhizome of an erect, unbranched perennial plant with leaves deeply divided and toothed, pink-to-purple flowers giving way to an elongated 'beaked' capsule; the rhizomes are sold in lengths of 2-10cm, dark-brown in colour, brittle, the upper surface with bud and stem scars, the lower covered with root scars; the taste is astringent.

Habitat: woodlands over North America.

Constituents: gallitannins.

Actions: astringent.

Applications: to control the symptoms of diarrhoea, and to reduce intestinal inflammations, as in peptic ulceration, enteritis and bowel disease (gentle enough to be used for the very young, the elderly and infirm); locally, as a mouthwash and gargle for disorders of the mouth, gums and throat, and as a douche for vaginal affections.

Dosage: 1-3 grams of dried rhizome equivalent three times per day.

Crataegus oxyacanthoides et spp, hawthorn.

Crohn's disease, an inflammatory and ulcerated condition of the lower small intestine, similar in many ways to **ulcerative colitis.** Although distinguished from the latter, treatment should be along similar lines.

---

croup, a spread and exacerbation of a cold to affect the larynx, possibly as part of a wider and more serious involvement of the rest of the respiratory system: it is most often found in children. As far as the croup itself is concerned it may be treated as for **laryngitis.**

---

cudweed, marsh, Cottonweed, Low cudweed, *Gnaphalium uliginosum* L. Fam: Compositae.

A branched, woolly annual plant less than 15cm high with narrow leaves, the upper with wavy edges; a tuft of longer leaves at branch tip encloses a cluster of small yellowish flowers.

Habitat: in waste places, especially farmyards and gateways, throughout Britain, Europe, Asia and northern North America.

Constituents: not known, a little volatile oil, probable tannins.

Actions: toning respiratory mucosa; anti-inflammatory.

Applications: to catarrhal conditions, especially of the pharynx and larynx, both systemically and as a gargle; effective for tonsillitis and quinsy.

Dosage: 1-4 grams of the dried herb equivalent three times per day.

---

curled dock, Yellow dock, Narrow-leafed dock, *Rumex crispus* L. Fam: Polygonaceae.

The root of one of a familiar group of species; the identifying characteristics are the narrowness of the leaves, with usually a curliness of the long edges, and the deep yellow colour of the root when scraped.

Habitat: in arable farmland, on roadsides, in ditches and waste places throughout the world.

Constituents: anthraquinone glycosides, tannins, bitter principles, resin, iron.

Actions: a mild laxative and cholagogue.

Applications: to chronic inflammatory conditions marked by sluggishness in the bowel or hepatic disturbance: particularly for skin conditions.

Dosage: 1-4 grams of dried root equivalent three times per day.

Cynara scolymus, artichoke, globe.

Cypripedium pubescens, lady's slipper.

---

cystitis, *see* **urinary infections.**

D

---

damiana, *Turnera diffusa var. aphrodisiaca* Urb. Fam: Turneraceae.

The stems and leaves of a shrub up to 2 metres high; the small leaves pale yellow-green with toothed margins and furred undersides; thin reddish-brown stems are found in commercial samples, along with occasional small yellow flowers that grow in the upper leaf axils; the aroma is strong and pleasant.

Habitat: indigenous to Texas, Mexico and Central America in humid conditions.

Constituents: volatile oil (including alpha- and beta-pinene, cineol, arbutin, cymene); alkaloids; bitter (damianin); flavonoid; cyanogenic glycoside; tannins; resins.

Actions: testosteromimetic action providing a generally stimulating and enhancing influence on those functions related to the reproductive system, especially in the male; also a mild laxative; nervous restorative.

Applications: to sexual inadequacies with a strong psychological or emotional element; to depression and debilitated states in both sexes.

Dosage: 1-4 grams of dried herb equivalent three times per day.

---

dandelion leaf, Pise-en-lit, Lion's tooth, Fairy clock, *Taraxacum officinale* Weber., *T. dens-leonis* Desf. Fam: Compositae.

A very well-known plant with characteristic 'lion's tooth' leaves, in a rosette from the centre of which arises the hollow stem bearing the yellow capitulate flowerhead giving way to the familiar 'fairy-clock'; the whole plant produces a milky-white sap when cut.

Habitat: originating in Central Asia, but now almost everywhere in the world, preferring moist positions, but clearly very adaptable.

Constituents: bitter glycosides, sterols, waxy substances, tannins, high levels of vitamins and minerals, notably potassium.

Actions: an effective but gentle diuretic, having sufficient potassium to make up for that leached out of the body in the diuretic process; hepatic and digestive tonic (but see the root below).

Applications: to oedema, especially of cardiac origin and as a natural complement to cardioactive remedies for failing heart; to urinary problems in general, especially where worsened by the presence of oliguria; to a lesser extent the same actions as the root (below).

Dosage: 4-10 grams of dried leaf equivalent three times per day.

---

dandelion root, *see above.*

The long taproot of the plant described above, also producing a white sap when cut.

Actions: digestive and hepatic tonic, cholagogue, diuretic and laxative.

Applications: as a supremely gentle tonic for liver function in a wide-range of problems (accepting that this organ has particular metabolic strains put on it in modern times — due to universal adulteration of the environment); gallstone and biliary problems; hepatic and post-hepatic jaundice; congestive dyspepsia with constipation; general toxic conditions such as chronic joint and skin inflammations; to a lesser extent, as for the leaf above; locally: the white sap may be applied directly for the long-term reduction of warts.

Dosage: 2-8 grams of dried root equivalent three times per day.

---

dandruff, the result of bacterial decomposition of the natural oil secreted from the hair follicles; a form of seborrheic eczema. Exacerbated by wearing hats, using sharp combs or brushes, and detergent shampoos (medicated shampoos often store up trouble for the future). Quillaia bark infusion is an excellent way of keeping the scalp clean, or soap spirit can be made by adding 1 litre of 90 per cent alcohol to 650 grams of soft soap: in all cases the scalp should be washed very thoroughly afterwards. Spirit or bay rum may be applied daily without washing. Internal treatment may be necessary, using **alteratives,** and digestive remedies as indicated; the diet should be low in fats and refined carbohydrates, high in fresh fruit and vegetables.

Datura stramonium, jimson weed.

Daucus carota, carrot, wild.

---

deadly nightshade, Belladonna, *Atropa belladonna* L. Fam: Solanaceae.

The leaf or root of an erect branching herb with perennial rootstock; stalked large ovate leaves are each usually coupled with a much smaller one; solitary flowers occur on short stalks in the axils of leaves, giving rise to violet-black large globular berries.

Habitat: waste and stony ground in southern Europe and west central Asia, extending over central Europe and southern Britain, probably as remains of earlier cultivation.

Constituents: alkaloids (including hyoscyamine, hyoscine and belladonnine).

Actions: anticholinergic activity, for example reducing spasm in the bronchi, gut wall, gall-bladder and urinary tract; central nervous depressant; locally analgesic (the root especially).

Applications: asthma; colic of the bowel, urinary system and gall-bladder; reducing excessive perspiration and salivation; in severe enuresis; reducing the symptoms of Parkinsonism.

Dosage: Maximum permitted dose is 50 mg of dried herb, 30mg of dried root equivalent three times per day.

Caution: this is a very toxic remedy which, in the United Kingdom, cannot be sold to anyone other than professional practitioners; its side effects include dry mouth, difficulty in swallowing, pupil dilation, slowing of the heart and respiration, confusion, delirium, coma and death. It must never be used in pregnancy, prostatic disease, tachycardia, glaucoma or with depressant drugs.

---

decoction, a preparation made by boiling remedies in water. Generally necessary when trying to extract from denser plant materials like roots, bark and woody samples (although if adequately ground down these may be infused, *see* **infusion**). Traditionally the technique involved boiling the plant and water mixture until the total volume was reduced by a third, then cooling and straining. However, loss of volatile elements is much reduced if the preparation is made in a modern 'slow-cooker' or 'crock-pot', where the temperature is kept below boiling point: in this case a cooking time of between 6 and 10 hours will be necessary. After straining and, if necessary, pressing, the liquid will keep only for a few days, and that in a refrigerator (*see* **tincture**).

demulcents, remedies which have a notable soothing effect on the membranes to which they are applied; generally a property of **mucilages** and **saponins,** and to a lesser extent **tannins** but *see* **astringent**). The demulcent remedies are applied to wounds, skin inflammations, and inflammation of the mouth, throat, oesophagus, stomach, vagina and any other accessible surface; their effect is primarily soothing, although many remedies have incidental healing or astringent properties which are enhanced by their demulcent properties. Whilst their local action is readily explicable as the physical effect of 'sliminess', their effects when taken internally are less obvious: thus they often have a pronounced effect on the respiratory system and urinary tract, as well as their expected action in reducing the symptoms of gut wall irritation: such effects can all in fact be explained as arising by reflex from soothing excitable gut wall membranes, via established embryonic neural links. Each remedy has a slightly different property in all these areas that depends on the actual physical properties of the relevant constituents, but notable examples of the group are chickweed, slippery elm, marshmallow, comfrey, Iceland moss, Irish moss, linseed, coltsfoot, meadowsweet, mullein, lungwort, psyllium, plantain, ribwort, fenugreek and white pond lily.

dental problems, tooth decay and **gum disease** are problems of modern diets and correction of abuses here are primary; it is illegal in the United Kingdom for unqualified persons to provide any treatment usually performed by dentists, and it is in any case doubtful that herbal measures will be effective in treating tooth decay. It is quite possible that mouthwashes will be helpful as prophylactics, and they may be used with great advantage in **gum problems**.

depression, seen in traditional herbal terms as a much wider debility than just the narrow nervous system (in classical terms, depression was seen as a problem of 'black bile': thus melancholia). It will thus usually be found that help is required on a number of fronts in any case, and attention should especially be directed to digestive and eliminative functions. As far as the nervous debility is concerned, **nervous restoratives** are indicated, to be applied consistently for weeks or months for slow but real improvement. (*See also* **nervous problems**.)

---

depurative, *see* **eliminative remedies.**

---

detoxification, a term sometimes used to describe the process of removing accumulated waste products, metabolites or chemical toxins from the body; normal detoxification is performed principally by the liver (but to a lesser extent most tissues), with elimination from the body through bile, bowel, kidney, lungs and sweat glands. In traditional, natural and naturopathic medicine, many chronic disease states are interpreted as either failure of one or other function, or overwhelming of the functions by dietary or drug excesses, or exposure to pollutants or toxins. Appropriate remedies are included within the following categories: **alterative, eliminative** and **hepatic.**

---

devil's claw, *Harpagophytum procumbens* D.C. Fam: Pedaliaceae.
 The tuber of a prostrate perennial plant with a long thick taproot (up to 1.5 metres) giving off secondary roots bearing the large bulbous tubers; above ground the plant is represented by prostrate shoots up to 1.5 metres long, bearing violet-to-red foxglove-like flowers, these giving way to horrendously spiked and barbed fruits; the tuber is sold in discs up to 6cm across.
 Habitat: in desert areas of Namibia, Botswana, and northern South Africa.
 Constituents: iridoid glycosides (harpagoside and harpagide).
 Actions: anti-inflammatory and analgesic (possible effects on hepatic and lymphatic functions).
 Applications: rheumatic and other joint disease; inflammation of connective tissues (e.g., myalgia, fibrositis, tendinitis).
 Dosage: 0.1-0.25 gram of the dried tuber equivalent three times per day.

---

diabetes mellitus, a condition of excessive levels of sugar in the blood brought about by progressive inability of the pancreas to secrete the hormone insulin on demand.

Generally divided into two groups: the more active 'juvenile onset' form that tends to occur in the young, and possibly results from an auto-immune destruction of the beta-cells in the pancreas that secrete insulin; and the more gradual 'late onset' type that may be characterized as a progressive exhaustion of the same cells. The former group will tend to have to rely on insulin injections to survive and, in most cases, are not amenable to herbal or other conservative treatment because of the risk of destabilizing the relationship with the insulin. The latter group are much more easily helped, at least in the early stages (it must be said however that no decision about diabetes must be made without qualified advice from a well-trained practitioner). The main aim in late-onset diabetes is to reduce the strain on the beta-cells, by reducing the rate at which glucose is absorbed from food: the simplest way is to provide high levels of roughage in the diet, in the form of wholegrains, pulses, vegetables and fruit, as such food tends to 'hang on' to its glucose, reducing the glucose surge into the bloodstream and the strain on insulin production. In many clinics, diabetes is controlled almost entirely by diet (*see also* **hypoglycaemia**); however, there are a number of other agents that will help keep excessive sugar levels down. They include goat's rue, garlic, the **bitters,** fenugreek, and such foods as cranberry, coconut, the brassicas, lettuce, spinach and carrot. All refined carbohydrates, alcohol, caffeine, should be strictly controlled.

---

diaphoretic, a remedy that promotes sweating; most examples actually produce an observable diaphoresis only when the body is in a feverish state, but it has traditionally been in this period when sweating has been seen as desirable (*see* **fever management**). Most diaphoretic remedies are also **peripheral vasodilators** and seem to stimulate the sweat glands in part by dilating the blood vessels in the area (although blood supply to the sweat glands themselves is controlled by a different mechanism from that controlling the remainder of peripheral blood flow). Notable diaphoretics include yarrow, vervain, elderflowers, limeflowers, hyssop, boneset, cinchona, ephedra, peppermint, rosemary, queen's delight, stone root, wood sage, ginger, galanga, snake root and blessed thistle. In traditional terms diaphoresis was seen as an eliminatory process, and it is known that the sweat glands perform in a rather crude way something of the function of the kidney nephrons; in other words sweating can be seen as augmenting or even substituting for kidney function; in fever, the onset of sweating, whether unaided or as a response to a diaphoretic herb, was seen as a cleansing operation, removing the toxic and other debris of the battle.

---

diarrhoea, frequency and looseness of the bowels; arises from any condition that irritates the gut wall along any part of its length and should be seen in the first place as a healthy cleansing response, not to be completely suppressed except in exceptional cases. Can be due to a passing difficulty in digestion, or to infection (**gastro-enteritis, food poisoning, dysentery,** typhoid, etc.), **food allergies** or other sensitivities, or possibly **ulcerative colitis, Crohn's disease, diverticulitis** or even **cancer.** It may also mark a **nervous bowel** where the condition is an irritability of the bowel muscle wall. Diarrhoea is potentially life-threatening, especially in children (most deaths in the Third World are due to diarrhoea in children) because of fluid and potassium depletion. Thus the condition, if unduly extended or severe, will need controlling to reduce danger. Herbal **astringents** are ideal for this purpose. Fluid and potassium may be replaced with plenty of drinks and, in spite of apparent paradox, by fruit and vegetables; *in extremis* by sugar and sea salt solutions. The underlying cause of any diarrhoea must always be actively investigated, and referral to a qualified practitioner is essential in any acute case.

---

digestive tonic, a remedy that appears to aid the processes of digestion; the **bitters** are the most prominent members of this group, but there are many herbs with a more warming character, that are most appropriate where digestive debility is part of a general chilled, run down or cachexic condition. Examples of such remedies are angelica, cardamom, celery, cinnamon, elecampane, fenugreek, galanga, ginger, golden seal, juniper, lovage, Oregon grape, parsley, sweet flag, thyme and yarrow.

---

dill, *Anethum graveolens* L. Fam: Umbelliferae.

The fruit of a tall biennial (up to 1.2 metres) with light feathery foliage with short leaf sheaths and umbels of yellow flowers; the fruit is brown to yellow-brown, in a lens shape with three dorsal ridges, the lateral two extended to wings; the odour and taste is strong and characteristic.

Habitat: indigenous to the Mediterranean regions but cultivated and naturalized widely elsewhere.

Constituents: volatile oil (including carvone and limonene).

Actions: carminative

Applications: to flatulence and colic (particularly useful for infants) and as an adjunct to laxatives and other medicines that might cause griping.

Dosage: 1-4 grams of dried fruits equivalent three times per day.

Dioscorea villosa, wild yam.

---

diuretic, a remedy that provokes an increase in the flow of urine; may work in one or more of a number of ways, but there are two basic groups: those that increase blood flow to the kidneys, and those that reduce the reabsorption of water from the filtrate in the kidney nephrons. In the former group are all **circulatory stimulant** and **cardioactive** remedies, and those containing caffeine (like kola, mate, coffee and tea). The latter group is the most diverse; most vegetable material is diuretic because several plant constituents are excreted via the kidneys and these act osmotically to bring more water with them: some remedies like couch grass and corn silk are notably effective in this regard, it is likely that most particularly diuretic herbs act in something of the same fashion, although some with high **volatile oil, saponin** or **alkaloid** content may irritate the reabsorption mechanism in some way. Diuretic remedies are used to reduce problems of **urinary infections** and **urinary stones,** to increase the loss of water in oedematous problems (and as an adjunct to **cardioactive** remedies in dropsy), and as part of an eliminatory programme. Apart from the remedies so far mentioned, notable diuretics include dandelion leaves, parsley piert, pellitory, parsley, celery, wild carrot, asparagus, birch, horsetail, juniper, gravel root, cleavers, broom, seven barks, stone root, ash, eryngo, heather flowers, and kava-kava. All stimulating **laxatives** are incidentally diuretic as well.

---

diverticulitis, the inflammation of small pouches arising in the weakened wall of the large bowel, perhaps due to the lodging of a pip or other particle; marked by pain and bowel irregularity. Pouches or diverticuli often form after a history of constipation or straining at stool and such causes should be seen to as a priority. Diet should be of high roughage but avoid items that may lodge in diverticuli, like pips, seeds, nuts, pears, celery, beans and soft fruit (apples and seedless grapes are ideal fruits to take). Pure bran may be too irritating as a source of roughage and should be replaced by proprietary gel preparations. Herbal treatment should be with **mucilages** and **astringents** and notably with comfrey and garlic.

---

dong quai, Tang kuei, Danggui, *Angelica senensis* (Oliv.) Diels. Fam: Umbelliferae.

The root of a herb of up to 1 metre in height with graceful spreading bipinnate leaves and large umbels; the tuberous taproot and long-spreading branch roots are obtained whole or sliced; it is characteristically aromatic and slightly sweet in taste.

Habitat: in high ground in cool and damp areas in western and north-western China.

Constituents: volatile oil (including carvacrol, safrol, n-dodecanol); sesquiterpenes; furanocoumarins; angelic acid; angelicone.

Actions: warming and sustaining to the circulation; regulating menstrual disorders; antispasmodic; alterative.

Applications: to painful, irregular or scanty menstrual periods, especially where accompanied by cramping and neuromuscular tension and/or debility, weakness or anaemia; to fleeting muscle and joint pains, especially when made worse by damp conditions; to dry and tense constipation.

Dosage: 2-6 grams of dried root equivalent three times per day.

Dorema ammoniacum, ammoniac.

---

douches, an aqueous solution directed against a part of the body or into a body cavity either for cleansing or antiseptic purposes; most often applied to **vaginal problems,** but the term includes eyebaths and nose washes.

Drosera rotundifolia, sundew.

---

drug addiction, the process of recovering from a period of addictive drug taking can be helped a great deal by the use of herbs; primary aims are to detoxify the system and to provide enough restorative stimulation that the need for false props can be progressively reduced. Detoxification is achieved principally by the use of **hepatic** remedies, **cholagogues** and **laxatives,** although **expectorants** and **alteratives** may also be indicated. Positive support may be provided with **circulatory stimulants** and **nervous restoratives,** with discretionary use of such stimulants as kola, damiana, Asiatic and Siberian ginseng; gotu kola has a number of useful benefits in this connection.

---

dysentery, inflammation and ulceration of the lower bowel with the painful passage at very frequent intervals of watery, slimy and bloody stools and often fever. May occur in a non-infective form (*see* **ulcerative colitis**) but more typically as either a bacillary or amoebic infection. The latter is confined entirely to tropical and sub-tropical countries and necessitates careful drug therapy (often with an alkaloid from the plant ipecacuanha): often follow-up treatment for liver involvement with herbal remedies (*see* **hepatics**) may be desirable. Bacillary dysentery is a form of **food poisoning** that may be contracted anywhere; it should initially be treated with conventional drugs, rest and a medium-fibre diet. Aftercare with garlic, **bitters** and healing remedies is recommended.

---

dyspepsia, a disturbance of digestion, marked by symptoms of nausea, heartburn, stomach congestion or discomfort, wind, occasional vomiting, all associated with taking food. May simply be due to excess intake of rich food or alcohol, or may denote a stressful or debilitated condition. Herbal **mucilages** and **astringents,** notably meadowsweet, comfrey, Iceland moss and marigold may be applied with effect, as can **relaxants** such as chamomile and lemon balm where tension is a factor, **carminatives** such as peppermint, cinnamon, fennel, thyme and ginger as appropriate, and **bitters** if there is evidence of sluggish digestion or overconsumption. If the dyspepsia is chronic it may be a sign of **gastritis, ulcers, gall-bladder disease, hepatitis** or **cancer,** but may equally be none of these things. Expert diagnosis is essential. *See also* **hyperacidity.**

E

---

ear problems, of the three chambers of the ear, practical treatment is only possible for the outer ear (or ear canal) and the middle ear containing the small ear bones and connecting by the Eustachian tube to the throat. The inner ear, containing the sense and balance organs is not generally accessible to herbal treatment (but *see* **travel sickness**). Infections, inflammations and irritation in the outer ear, as well as catarrhal problems of the middle ear (on the other side of the ear drum), can be profitably treated with ear drops. In most cases olive oil or similar is used as a vehicle: to this may be added such agents as garlic and mullein flowers for middle ear problems, and marigold, comfrey or chickweed for local problems in the canal. Excessive wax production is treated by daily drops of warmed olive oil so that any impacted plug can be softened for removal by syringing (practitioners only); the canal may then be washed with an aqueous solution of tormentil root or witch hazel with marigold. Before any ear drops are applied it is necessary to be sure that the ear drums are undamaged: a practitioner will confirm this if necessary. Catarrhal conditions of the middle ear or Eustachian tube, often giving earache, especially in young children, should be seen as variations of upper respiratory catarrh (*see* **catarrh**). Apart from such internal medication as is appropriate, inhaling steam and volatile oils will be found to be especially useful.

---

echinacea, Purple coneflower, Rudbeckia, Black samson, *Echinacea angustifolia* (DC) Heller., *E. pallida* (Nutt) Britt. Fam: Compositae.

The root and rhizome of a perennial herb 60-100 cm in height with simple rough stems, hollow near the base and thickening slightly close to the flowerhead; the leaves are elongated, slightly elliptical with entire margins and covered with coarse hairs and protruberances; the purple flower is in the form of a high cone surrounded by rough hairy bracts, downturned purple ray florets and greenish tubular florets; the tapering root is greyish-brown flecked with white, with an aromatic odour, and a taste which is first sweet, then bitter, leaving a tingling sensation on the tongue.

Habitat: the prairies of the western U.S.A. and as a cultivated ornamental plant in Europe.

Constituents: volatile oil, glycoside (echinacoside), echinacein, acetylenes, resin.

Actions: anti-infective, increasing the body's resistance to infections; stimulating, warming alterative, inhibits hyaluronidase activity; reduces eosinophil levels.

Applications: to septic and infected conditions, furunculosis, tonsillitis, abscesses, pyorrhoea, etc., especially where chronic and marked by debility and cold; to improving resistance to and recovery from all infections, viral and fungal as well as bacterial; particularly applicable to low-grade subclinical infections of the salpinges, lungs and other visceral structures, and to the chronic inflammatory diseases resulting from these; locally as a mouthwash, douche and lotion for appropriate infections.

Dosage: 0.5-1 gram of the dried root equivalent three times per day.

Echinacea angustifolia et spp., echinacea.

---

eczema, an inflammatory reaction of the skin tissues to an internal or external irritant, marked by rashes, spots, blisters, exfoliation, thickening and drying ('dry eczema') or weeping and discharging ('weeping eczema'). External causes tend to produce eczema on sites exposed to the irritant, e.g., hands in those sensitive to washing detergents or cement, around rings, watchstraps or bra straps in those sensitive to nickel (as in stainless steel); withdrawal of the irritant usually leads to a quick improvement. Some external irritants are more difficult to pin down, and may cause widespread eczema over the body (especially airborne irritants): a considerable amount of detective work is often necessary. Having discovered a cause it is still desirable to encourage the body to be less sensitive to the material: the procedure for this is much the same as when dealing wholly with internal causes. These may come in any form. Nervous and emotional tension is certainly exacerbatory and **relaxant** remedies are often indicated, especially in children. Poor eliminations are likely factors, and **eliminative** remedies will be chosen as appropriate, along with **alterative** herbs (these two groups are those most favoured in traditional treatments of eczema). Increasingly today a search should be conducted for possible **food allergies,** and appropriate measures taken: if in doubt about this it is simply sufficient to see how the eczema fares with a much reduced choice of foods for a week or so. Food allergies are particularly likely to be major factors in infantile or juvenile eczema, and cow's milk should be most exhaustively checked. For external problems such as itching soothing applications of herbs may be applied, *see* **pruritus.**

---

elder, Black Elder, *Sambucus nigra* L. Fam: Caprifoliaceae.
The flowers of the familiar shrubby tree with stiff pithy stems and smooth segmented and toothed leaves; the powerfully aromatic inflorescences of white flowers appear in early summer, giving way to purple-red berries.
Habitat: along hedgerows, in woods and wasteplaces throughout all northern temperate regions.
Constituents: volatile oil, flavonoids (including rutin), tannins, mucilage.
Actions: gentle circulatory stimulant with a strong diaphoretic effect in the feverish patient; expectorant and anticatarrhal; diuretic; locally anti-inflammatory.
Applications: to feverish conditions especially where involving the lungs and respiratory system (e.g., influenza); catarrhal problems in general, especially where associated with cold; as a mouthwash and gargle for mouth and throat inflammations.
Dosage: 2-4 grams of dried flowers equivalent three times a day; best

results are obtained with fresh or frozen flowers at up to three times the weight per dose.

---

elecampane, Elfwort, Scabwort, *Inula helenium* L. Fam: Compositae. The roots of a large herbaceous perennial, with stiff robust stems 0.5-2 metres high, having at their base large elliptical hairy leaves, and supporting corymbs of 2-3 flowerheads 6-8cm in diameter, bright yellow in colour. The odour of the dried roots is characteristically aromatic.

Habitat: native of south-east Europe and western Asia, but found as a naturalized escape in Britain, Ireland and north mid-west U.S.A.

Constituents: volatile oil ('helenin' — including camphor and related constituents), bitter principles, triterpenoid saponins, mucilage.

Actions: a stimulating **expectorant,** diaphoretic, digestive tonic, relaxant, warming, bacteriostatic.

Applications: to congestive bronchial and pulmonary conditions and to helping the cough arising out of such conditions by increasing its productivity; applicable especially to chronic bronchitic problems in the elderly; for different reasons also useful in congestive complaints in children; traditionally indicated for the cough of pulmonary tuberculosis; can be relied on to support a debilitated constitution and digestion.

Dosage: 1-4 grams of dried root equivalent three times a day.

Eleutherococcus senticosus, ginseng, Siberian.

---

eliminative, a remedy that encourages one or more of the body's eliminatory functions; the purpose of using such an agent is to increase the removal of metabolites and toxic material from the body, a measure that has always been an important part of the herbalist's approach to illness; in these terms many diseases, especially those of a chronically inflamed nature (such as skin, arthritic and **auto-immune** diseases, and **cancer**) are primarily of a toxic nature, and there is likely to be a toxic factor in almost any circumstances; toxicity is seen as an accumulation of cell waste products and ingested toxins, either as a result of an inadequate eliminatory function, poor tissue circulation, poor liver function, poor digestion, or excessive ingestion of chemicals, additives, adulterants or other toxins. It is accepted in orthodox pathological terms that many metabolites and other agents can produce significant changes in tissue function, but herbalists have traditionally made more of this feature than allopathic medicine. In each case therefore, likely departures from tissue 'cleanliness' are assessed from circumstantial or direct clinical evidence, and where appropriate one or more of the following groups of herbs may be employed: **laxatives, lymphatics, expectorants, diuretics, cholagogues** (traditionally **emetics**) and, in fever, **diaphoretics;** it may also be appropriate to use **digestive tonics** or **hepatics;** quite often it is necessary to concentrate on a focus of infection, whether with **anti-infectives,** or in a local accessible position (notably throat or mouth, a major trouble spot) appropriate **antiseptic** remedies. *See also* **alteratives.**

---

elixir,   a flavoured liquid preparation of herbs or other medicines, often with a lot of sugar.

Elletaria cardamomum,   cardamom.

---

embrocation,   a form of **liniment.**

---

emetic,   a remedy that induces vomiting; once a very frequent part of the traditional herbalist's treatment but very much less used in developed societies today. Easily rejected as crude and of limited use, the emetic not only cleared out the contents of the stomach but, when expertly applied, provided one of the few ways of clearing bile from the body effectively (a large part of it is reabsorbed in its passage down through the gut under normal circumstances); it also provides for possibly the most effective reflex cleansing of congested lung contents as well. Nevertheless, the use of emetics was confined to those with the most robust constitution as the process is quite an exhausting one: it is an unfortunate fact that few people in modern civilized society would fit the standards of robustness accepted as widespread in more primitive conditions. Remedies that produce emesis when used in large enough doses include ipecacuanha, lobelia, squills, snake root, bryony and queen's delight. Many of these when used in sub-emetic doses are stimulating **expectorants** (*see also* **vomiting**).

---

emmenogogue,   a remedy that promotes menstruation; formerly applied to remedies that brought on delayed menstruation, or that in other words were **abortifacients** in the overwhelming majority of cases; it is thus inadvisable to use the term freely, as is often the case in popular herb books, as synonymous with a gynaecological remedy; *see instead* **uterine remedies,**

hormonal remedies, menstrual disorders, menopause and other specific conditions.

---

emollient, a term descriptive of remedies that soothe the surface to which they are applied; *see* **demulcent.**

---

enemas, an administration of liquid medicines via the rectum, either to promote a bowel movement, to treat a local bowel inflammation or infection or to provide the body with internal medication, absorbed without being subject to the metabolizing effect of the liver. The fluid is generally applied, at varying volumes, with special apparatus and with great care; the main dangers lie in unduly altering the bacterial flora of the bowel, and in presenting the system with a large load of material readily absorbed into the body fluids.

---

ephedra, Ma-Huang, *Ephedra sinica* Stapf., *E. equisetina* Bunge., and *E. gerardiana* Wall. Fam: Ephedraceae.

The young stems of three species of perennial herbs, obtained in broom-like tufts of slender green stems arising in bunches of twenty or so out of more woody older stems; they may be up to 30cm long, with nodes every 1-6cm and leaves reduced to sheaths surrounding the stems; the taste is bitter and acrid, the odour strong and aromatic.

Habitat: northern China; *E. gerardiana* from India.

Constituents: alkaloids (including ephedrine, methyl ephedrine, norephedrine).

Actions: warming peripheral vasodilator and diaphoretic; bronchial relaxant; both alpha- and beta-adrenergic action so some cardiac stimulation; diuretic.

Applications: to bronchial spasm in asthma and other hypersensitivities; to cold conditions affecting the chest, with chills, aching, fever without sweating, and breathlessness; where any such conditions above are linked with water retention.

Dosage: maximum permitted is 0.6 grams of dried stems equivalent three times per day; recommended initial dose is 50-100mg.

Caution: although the toxicity of the whole herb is not clearly established it is controlled in the U.K. under the terms of the Medicines Act 1968 so that it is available only to practitioners; official precautions (linked with evidence for ephedrine in isolation, *not* for the whole herb) are to avoid it in severe hypertension, glaucoma, hyperthyroidism and coronary thrombosis, or together with MAOI anti-depressants. It would be wise to observe these.

Ephedra sinica et spp, ephedra.

---

epilepsy, condition resulting from disturbances in brain function with attacks graded by severity into 'grand mal' and 'petit mal' forms. Full treatment is unlikely and it is in practice usually necessary to rely on one or other anti-epileptic drug, especially in cases of grand mal. It is possible however to help contain any epileptic condition with such remedies as scullcap.

Equisetum arvense, horsetail.

Eryngium maritimum, eryngo.

---

eryngo, Eringo, Sea holly, *Eryngium maritimum* L. Fam: Umbelliferae.
The roots of a stiff erect branched perennial plant up to 30 cm high with smooth bluish-grey foliage and broad, stiff, sinuous leaves divided into three broad lobes, prominently veined and bordered by coarse prickly teeth; the flowerheads are characteristic blue and globular.
Habitat: on sandy soil especially on sea coasts throughout Britain, Ireland, Europe and Asia.
Constituents: saponins.
Actions: diuretic, appearing to help reduce urinary stone formation.
Applications: to the symptoms of urinary calculi (pain, frequency, bleeding); prostatic inflammations.
Dosage: 1-4 grams of the dried root equivalent three times per day.

---

erysipelas, *see* **abscess.**

---

ethnopharmacology, the study of medicines used in **traditional medicine,** in order to find useful remedies for modern times; two main strands: (1) anthropological recording of remedies used, and (2) scientific investigation into the potential value of such plants. A significant feature in orthodox drug research but of major value to herbalism as well.

Eugenia jambolana,   jambul.

Eupatorium perfoliatum,   boneset.

Eupatorium purpureum,   gravel root.

---

euphorbia,   Pill-bearing Spurge, *Euphorbia hirta* L., *E. pilulifera* L. Fam: Euphorbiaceae.

An annual with slender hairy stem and lanceolate opposite-toothed leaves; small yellow flowers occur in dense clusters in the leaf axils producing small reddish wrinkled seeds; the plant produces a milky latex which is irritating to mucous membranes.

Habitat: India and most tropical countries.

Constituents: triterpenoids, sterols, alkaloid, glycoside, tannin.

Actions: antispasmodic and antiasthmatic; expectorant and anti-catarrhal.

Applications: asthmatic conditions and bronchial asthma.

Dosage: 0.1-0.3 gram of dried herb three times per day.

Euphorbia hirta et spp,   euphorbia.

Euphrasia officinalis,   eyebright.

---

expectorant,   a remedy that encourages the passage up the bronchial apparatus of phlegm and other material in the lung; there is a very ingenious 'mucociliary escalator' that normally brings bronchial secretions and adherent dust and other airborne matter up to the throat as phlegm or sputum, but in many respiratory conditions this self-cleansing process may be impeded or overloaded. There are two main types of problem: in the first an excessive mucous secretion (*see* **catarrh**) leads to overloading of the escalator with resulting congestion in the lung base (*see* **bronchitis, bronchiectasis, pneumonia**); in the second the mucous secretion is checked and/or thickened as part of an inflammatory, hypersensitivity or nervous reaction, to result in a tight, dry, irritable condition as seen in nervous, irritable, dry or tickly cough, or **asthma**. For the first, 'congestive', 'wet' or 'cold' condition, *'stimulating expectorants'* are indicated; these act to stimulate extraordinary activity in the escalator or lead to an even more productive cough; many of this group act principally as stimulants to the stomach wall (*see* **emetics** and **saponins**), which is thought to lead to a reflex stimulation of the bronchial apparatus. Examples of stimulating expectorants are as follows: elecampane, ipecacuanha, squill, cowslip, bittersweet, heartsease, (white) horehound, balm of Gilead, asafoetida, blood root, arbor-vitae, mouse-ear, queen's delight, rue, (wild) thyme, bryony, caraway, snake root and violet. For the 'dry', 'irritable', or 'hot' condition, *'relaxing expectorants'* are indicated: these are generally soothing on the upper digestive lining (*see* **demulcents, mucilages** *and* **volatile oils**) and appear to act by reflex to soothe bronchial spasm and loosen mucous secretions. Examples of relaxing expectorants include: coltsfoot, marshmallow, comfrey, plantain, ribwort, linseed, licorice, aniseed, lungwort, thyme, hyssop, grindelia, ephedra, pleurisy root, sundew, skunk cabbage, (sweet) chestnut, ammoniac, Irish moss and euphorbia. It is implicit in the above account that it would generally be inappropriate to use a relaxing expectorant for congestive bronchial conditions and stimulating expectorants for asthmatic or irritable coughs. There are however some remedies with a particularly broad-range effect which in different ways can be used where there is a complexity of symptoms: these include lobelia, garlic, ginger, mullein flowers, red clover, lovage and elderflowers.

---

expression, a process in manufacturing herbal medicines where the liquid is forced out of solid material by pressure; most often used to obtain juices from fresh plant material, as in the preparation of 'green extracts' and homoeopathic mother tinctures. The resultant juice is often referred to as a succus: it has very poor keeping qualities unless immediately mixed with alcohol or similar preservative.

---

extract, a preparation of a herb obtained by extraction in a suitable solvent, most often water (*see* **infusion, decoction**) or an alcohol/water mixture (*see* **tincture**); liquid or **fluid extracts** so-called are generally taken as extracts where the strength of one part by volume of the liquid is equivalent to one part by weight of the original herb, although there may be other more positive assessments of strength laid down in official pharmacopoeias; their production involves either an evaporation of surplus liquid to achieve the desired strength, or, more beneficially for the final preparation, repeated extractions by the same liquid of fresh herbal material. Solid extracts, so-called, are produced by the total evaporation of a tincture or fluid extract so as to leave a solid residue: it is of course a very concentrated form of the original agent, but there is also likely to be loss of volatile and other constituents in the process.

---

extraction, the processes by which soluble constituents of a herb are separated off in solution (*see* **extract**).

---

eyebright, *Euphrasia officinalis* L. *et spp.* Fam: Scrophulariaceae.
An extremely variable small bushy annual herb, though occasionally reaching 30cm in height, with small, sessile, deeply toothed leaves, the flowers in loose terminal leafy spikes, white or red and occasionally yellow, with purple streaks and a yellow spot in the throat.
Habitat: alpine pastures and other grassy places throughout Britain, Europe and Asia, naturalized locally in parts of the United States.
Constituents: glycosides (including aucubin), tannins, resins, volatile oil.
Actions: astringent and anti-inflammatory; anticatarrhal.
Applications: as an eyebath for conjunctivitis and other superficial eye inflammations; as a mouthwash and gargle for inflammations of the mouth and throat; systemically for watery catarrhal conditions of nose, sinus and middle ear.
Dosage: 1-4 grams of herb equivalent three times per day.

---

eye problems, in practice problems of the surface of the eye, conjunctiva and eyelids: internal problems such as cataracts, glaucoma, retinal problems and the various causes of blindness are not readily approached by herbal treatment, although there is always scope in any case for looking at the condition of the whole person. There is one problem, inflammation of the iris, or iritis, that may be seen as an extension of wider inflammatory disease, especially **auto-immune disease,** gonorrhoea, **diabetes** and **tuberculosis,** or even infection of teeth, gums, sinuses and throat: in as far as such conditions are treatable in their own right it may be possible to help the iritis indirectly. For more superficial problems, particularly conjunctivitis, inflammation of the eyelid (blepharitis), styes, or simple irritation, local eyebaths are applicable. Prime remedies are eyebright, fennel, licorice, marigold, raspberry leaves or chamomile, all prepared in decoction form (infusions may not sterilize the herb adequately). Many eye problems are secondary to other problems, such as **hay fever** and other allergies, **colds,** debility and general illness, and these will require primary attention. Styes may be considered as one would consider an attack of **boils.** Obviously exposure to smoke and other irritating causes should be restricted.

F

Fagopyrum esculentum, buckwheat.

false unicorn root, *see* **helonias root.**

febrifuge, remedy that reduces fever, *see* **fever management.**

fennel, *Foeniculum vulgare* (Mill) Thelung. Fam: Umbelliferae.
The fruit of an umbelliferous biennial 60-90cm high with finely dissected leaves with large flowering umbels eventually producing double fruits each with five longitudinal ridges, and with characteristic aroma.
Habitat: in dry rocky situations, especially in coastal areas, probably originally from southern Europe but possibly native to many coastal regions, including those of southern Britain; now found throughout Europe and Asia.
Constituents: volatile oil (including anethol and fenchone), bitter principle, fixed oil.
Actions: carminative; circulatory stimulants; anti-inflammatory; galactogogue; diuretic.
Applications: griping, colic, flatulence and other disturbances of bowel or intestinal function, particularly applied when there is inadequate digestive tone; locally, especially as an eyewash or gargle, for mucous membrane inflammations; to promote breast milk production.
Dosage: 200-600mg of dried fruit equivalent three times per day.

fenugreek, *Trigonella foenum-graecum* L. Fam: Leguminosae.

The seeds of an annual herb growing up to 60cm high with slender smooth stems and slim ovate trefoil leaves, the upper leaves supporting in their axils pale yellow leguminous flowers, giving way to sickle-shaped pods each containing 5-20 seeds; these are rhomboidal, yellow-brown, about 5-7mm long and 2mm thick; they have a strong odour like lovage, and a bitter taste.

Habitat: countries around the eastern Mediterranean and cultivated throughout the Middle East.

Constituents: steroidal saponin (diosgenin), alkaloid (trigonelline), bitter principle, mucilage, volatile oil.

Actions: nutritive and digestive tonic; galactogogue; hypoglycaemic; locally demulcent, healing and anti-inflammatory.

Applications: to debility and convalescence where digestion and nutrition are poor; gastric inflammation; to promote lactation; locally for skin inflammations and infections.

Dosage: 1-6 grams of dried seeds equivalent three times per day.

Ferula asa-foetida, asafoetida.

---

fever, the symptoms associated with a rise in body temperature (pyrexia), most often initiated in turn by an infection. In traditional medicine, fevers were by far the most common condition, and were also the main cause of death, from puerperal fever striking down women in childbirth, to the legion childhood fevers, now infrequent or mild, like diphtheria, measles or scarlet fever, and to the wide variety of others: smallpox, typhoid, cholera, pneumonia, whooping cough, poliomyelitis, pyelonephritis, rheumatic fever, mumps, glandular fever and influenza. Herbal remedies were in large part, therefore, geared toward dealing with fevers; although they were not responsible for eliminating the problem, herbal management of fevers, in expert hands at least, was clearly very effective. It can moreover be argued that much of the problem with fevers arose from the unhealthy environment and poor hygiene and public health measures of the day, and it has been shown that it was the improvement in such areas that led to a decline in the killer fevers even before the arrival of the antibiotics. Nowadays, using herbal remedies, with the support of antibiotics and other drugs where necessary, the prospects for fever sufferers are extremely good. Herbal treatment confers advantages specifically because it is geared to *helping the body through its fever.* Whereas drugs like aspirin simply 'switch off' the fever at source, and antibiotics kill the infecting organisms directly, both measures having no regard for the possible value of the fever response, the herbalist sees fever as a valuable opportunity to 'flex' the body's emergency defences, to *strengthen* the body if well done, and uses remedies that improve the performance of these defences. The aim is to shorten the fever by improving its efficiency, at the same time providing such remedies as will calm and reduce excessive symptoms associated with the struggle (*see* **fever management**). Some fevers are not infective in origin, or may pursue idiosyncratic courses, and it is necessary to be qualified in recognizing the complications and dangers before taking on all responsibility in any case. However, the most frequently used remedies are inherently safe and generously broad-based in their effects, so that it is quite possible to learn the basic techniques that valuably augment simple common nursing care.

---

feverfew, Featherfew, Midsummer daisy, *Tanacetum parthenium* (L) Schult. *Chrysanthemum parthenium* (L) Bernh., *Pyrethrum parthenium* Sm. Fam: Compositae.

The leaves of an erect perennial herb, 25-60cm in height, with yellowish to dark green relatively shiny leaves, heavily divided, and long-stalked chamomile-like flowerheads; the whole plant has a strong, characteristic camphor-like aroma (though not to be confused with tansy, which has all-yellow flowers).

Habitat: common to wasteland, field borders, etc., throughout central and southern Europe, Britain and many other places around the world; indigenous to the Balkans.

Constituents: sesquiterpene lactones (including parthenolide and santamarine), volatile oil, pyrethrin, tannins.

Actions: anti-inflammatory (salicylate-like antiprostaglandin activity); vasodilatory; relaxant; digestive stimulant; uterine stimulant.

Applications: to migraine headaches of a vasoconstrictory type (i.e., those relieved by applying heat to the head); arthritis in the active inflammatory stage; vertigo, tinnitus and other head disorders relieved by heat; to sluggish menstrual flow and congestive dysmenorrhoea; after labour to hasten cleansing and toning of the womb.

Dosage: the equivalent of one fresh leaf 1-3 times daily (best taken fresh, frozen or freeze-dried).

Caution: side-effects include mouth ulcers, and soreness of the mouth can occur; it is probably best avoided in pregnancy.

---

fever management, a central skill for the medical herbalist, one for which herbal remedies are well suited. The primary aim (*see* **fever**) is to improve the efficiency of the body's response to the intrusion or stress on its integrity whilst providing relief to the sufferer rather than simply suppressing the condition. The rise in temperature is seen as the principal mechanism in a mobilizing of the body's defence measures (particularly the white blood cells and immune system) and in practice a febrile temperature of around 101°-102°F (38°-39°C) is an ideal to be aimed for and held to (compared with a normal temperature of around 98.4°F or 37°C) as it is at this point that the odds are tipped most favourably against the disrupting influence. Typically a rising body temperature is marked by shivering and a feeling of cold ('chill') as the body perceives that its actual body temperature is 'too low.' for the new level set by the 'thermostat' of the hypothalamus in the brain. When the actual temperature is at the same level as the 'thermostat' the patient feels relatively comfortable (apart from other symptoms of the particular disease); when the temperature is falling, there is sweating and a feeling of heat, as the actual body temperature is too high for the re-set 'thermostat' level. Thus, armed with a clinical thermometer, it is possible to tell what the actual level is and whether it is likely to rise further or fall. If the temperature is too high or rising, then 'normalizing' remedies, those originally classified in Galenic terms as 'hot in the first degree', are appropriate. Notable examples are yarrow, boneset, elderflowers, vervain, limeflowers and hyssop, each with its own properties influencing the final choice, but all under some circumstances having a diaphoretic or sweat-inducing effect, in others a heating action: they are actually genuinely normalizing on body temperature, and selectively used (i.e., geared to results) they will help maintain an ideal temperature, for as long as is necessary. Where more positive cooling is required the 'cooling' remedies (those 'cold in the first degree') may be selected. Most of these are, in fact, **bitters** and their use is often additionally indicated, particularly as defective digestion is a frequent disruptive factor in fever. When it looks as though the temperature is rising to dangerous heights (i.e. over 105°F, 40.5°C) then drugs may be necessary to curtail the escalation, although the expert herbal practitioner will cope with most such cases. It may be, however, that the practitioner considers the fever response too sluggish (particularly in those debilitated, or past adolescent prime). In this case 'warming' or 'heating' remedies may be used (*see* **circulatory stimulants**). Those 'hot in the second degree' like angelica root, cinnamon, cassia, cardamom, lovage, garlic or echinacea may be used quite readily, according to indication, to support any flagging vitality; those 'hot in the third degree',such as ginger, horseradish and cayenne, need more care, but they provide the prospect of the most effective stimulus to the fever response (they will quite markedly raise body temperature). Maintaining a good temperature during fever will allow the body to tackle the intrusion most expeditiously and will hasten the resolution of the problem. It will often be necessary, however, to calm and comfort, to reduce distressing or debilitating symptoms associated with the particular condition. Thus **relaxants** are often indicated, **antispasmodics** occasionally so, **expectorants, bitter** tonics (*see above*), **anti-infective** remedies, **alteratives, diuretic** remedies, and **astringent** remedies to manage any diarrhoea are all likely to be used. The aim in all cases is to use such remedies as relieve and relax, rather than suppress, vital responses. (*See also* individual disease headings.) A fever, even one successfully negotiated, is an exhausting event for the body, and a proper programme of **convalescence,** with appropriate remedies, is an essential part of the treatment. Throughout any fever episode food intake should be restricted (an initial fast is often advisable) but fluid intake should be high.

fibroids, benign growths in the womb, generally, but not always, occurring in later reproductive life, and most often characterized by increasingly heavy periods, or even bleeding outside menstruation. Non-surgical removal or reduction of existing fibroids must be considered unlikely (most doctors would say impossible), but it is possible for fibroid-induced problems to be alleviated in some cases, and for further growth to be checked. Practitioners might choose from helonias root, blue cohosh, agnus-castus, damiana, life root, motherwort and black cohosh. They would also check for any possible predisposing condition, notably any signs of congestion in the pelvic area.

fibrositis, *see* **myalgia.**

figwort, Scrophula plant, Carpenter's square, *Scrophularia nodosa* L. Fam: Scrophulariaceae.
A coarse erect perennial plant with thick, sharply-square, fleshy stems 60-150cm in height, arising from a knotted horizontal rootstock; leaves are opposite, short-stemmed ovate at base, lanceolate near the top, with toothed margins; the flowers are in loose cymes in pyramidal or oblong panicles; each flower is globular, five green sepals encircling a green or purple flower, giving way to an egg-shaped seed capsule.
Habitat: moist and cultivated waste ground, in woodlands and copses throughout the northern hemisphere except western North America.

Constituents: saponins, cardioactive glycosides, flavonoids, anti-inflammatory glycosides.

Actions: alterative with circulatory stimulating properties; anti-inflammatory; diuretic and laxative.

Applications: to chronic inflammatory conditions, especially as affecting the skin and when marked by swollen lymph nodes; traditionally for discharging skin disease; a general alterative remedy at its best in conditions of poor circulation.

Dosage: 2-8 grams of dried herb equivalent three times per day.

Caution: to be avoided in tachycardia and other heart conditions.

Filipendula ulmaria, meadowsweet.

---

fissure, a cleft appearing in skin or mucous membrane, especially at the corners of the mouth, at the edge of the anus, and as part of eczema, on the hands and fingers. To be treated as an open wound or **ulcer,** with local healing herbs applied as poultices or other non-oily application. Often measures have to be taken to reduce daily strain on the area: for example, taking mucilaginous **laxatives** to bulk up and soften the stool to reduce straining in anal fissures.

---

fits, *see* **convulsions.**

---

flatulence, the production of gas by bowel contents or in the stomach; in the latter case the most common cause is unconscious air-swallowing, then dietary indiscretion, **gall-bladder disease** (usually associated with fats in the diet), and **gastritis,** nervous **dyspepsia, ulcer** or stomach cancer; bowel flatulence may be secondary to that in the stomach, or may follow fermentation of contents due to incomplete digestion (best treated with **bitter remedies), food allergies** or sensitivities, **constipation** or **nervous bowel,** or the excessive use of **laxatives.** It is best in all cases to attempt to find and treat background causes, but flatulence may be helped directly by **carminatives,** with particular attention paid to the most warming in character, e.g., cayenne, ginger, cinnamon, cardamom, aniseed or fennel.

---

flavonoid glycosides, yellow-coloured phenols found very commonly in plants, with sweet or bitter taste, but with interesting pharmacological properties: most are **diuretic,** some are **antispasmodic, anti-inflammatory** and **antiseptic** in isolation and it is likely that they contribute to such effects in the whole plant. Prominent flavonoids like rutin and citrin are well-known as 'bioflavonoids' in nutritional circles, and have a healing and toning effect on the walls of the peripheral blood vessels (*see* **vascular remedies).** Flavonoids are most likely to be found in white and yellow flowers, plants with yellow or red coloration, in citrus fruits, and in such herbs as buckwheat and rue.

---

fluid extract, or Liquid Extract, is the traditionally most popular method of providing herbal remedies commercially; it allows for a concentrated fluid form of the remedy most convenient for administering as a medicine. Its strength is stated as 1:1, that is, 1cc of the liquid is equivalent to 1 gram of the dried herb. Several techniques are used, including evaporation by heat in vacuum of a **tincture** and reconstituting with alcohol to the required strength, and cold percolation with alcohol/water solvent. The former is the most widely used but the resulting products have been criticized for the loss of volatile and other constituents (though many traditional practitioners have used these, and **decoctions,** with success); cold percolation is returning to favour in modern times.

Foeniculum vulgare,   fennel.

---

food allergies,   sensitivity, often masked, to constituents in the diet. Most common allergens are cow's milk, and foods containing the protein gluten (products of wheat, oats, rye and barley) but almost any food can contain an allergen, usually a protein; in general, the sensitivity arises through the intrusion of an undigested protein into the body fluids over and above the capacity of the immune system to deal with such invasion quietly. It tends to start either when digestion is defective (e.g., in infancy, anorexia nervosa, or in cases of digestive impairment), and at times when the body's defences are under stress. Typically the food concerned is taken frequently, for its ability to provide the secretion of stimulatory 'cover-up' hormones and thus to appear as a 'pick-me-up'. Trial eliminations of foods are the simplest way to check the possibility: such eliminations must be 100 per cent complete for the protein concerned and should last at least a week. Herbal treatment emphasizes the stimulation of digestion with **bitters,** and remedies that improve the integrity of the gut wall: **tannin**-containing remedies, marigold, golden seal, etc. Liver remedies are often indicated.

---

food poisoning, due to the consumption of chemical or natural poisons, or particular bacteria or their toxins. The symptoms are abdominal pain, diarrhoea and/or vomiting. They come quickly if poisons have been ingested, up to two days later for some bacterial food poisoning. The symptoms can be severe, and dangerous. Immediate referral must be made to medical attention, and notification of the outbreak is necessary to trace the source of contamination. Notable examples of bacterial poisoning are due to salmonella and include typhoid and paratyphoid. Botulism is a rare but most serious version. Where food poisoning is likely, as for example in some countries or in unhygienic eating conditions, it may largely be prevented by consuming the **bitters** and **hot spices,** which act to increase the protective barrier of stomach digestive juices and acid.

fractures, normal vital repair of bone breaks and fractures can be significantly stimulated by the local application of comfrey around the affected area (it is thought that the ready diffusion of its constituent allantoin through the tissues is at least partly responsible); unfortunately modern encasing plasters often prevent such local applications and oral administration may be tried; mouse-ear has a similar reputation.

Fraxinus excelsor, ash.

Fucus vesiculosus, kelp.

Fumaria officinalis, fumitory.

fumitory, Earth smoke, *Fumaria officinalis* L. Fam: Fumariaceae.
   A delicate annual herb with fine, erect, ridged stems 15-30cm high, or higher when it becomes decidedly straggly; the fine leaves are three-lobed and stalked; the delicate pink-purple flowers with darker tips appear on flowering shoots growing from axils of small bracts.
   Habitat: common throughout Europe on cultivated and waste land, though native to the Mediterranean regions.
   Constituents: alkaloids (including protopine, fumarine); bitter principles; mucilage; resin.
   Actions: antispasmodic; choleretic; laxative; diuretic.
   Applications: as a 'blood-cleanser' particularly applied to chronic skin

diseases especially in any condition where liver or bile disturbances seem significant; for migraine under similar conditions; to calm biliary colic in gall-bladder disease.

Dosage: 1-4 grams of dried herb equivalent three times per day.

G

galactogogue, a remedy that promotes lactation or the flow of milk from the breast. Examples that may safely be tried include: fennel, fenugreek, nettle, vervain, celery and cleavers.

galanga, Galangal, Chinese ginger, Colic root, *Alpinia officinarium* Hance. Fam: Zingiberaceae.

The rhizome of a perennial herb growing up to 1.6 metres in height with reed-like leaves and a flower spike terminating in white flowers; the rhizome is obtained as hard branching pieces covered in red-brown cork, with a greyish-brown cut surface with numerous red resin cells; the odour is pungent and spicy, with spicy taste, reminiscent of ginger.

Habitat: indigenous to Hainan Island, off China, and Java.

Constituents: volatile oil, galangol, methyl cinnamate, galangine, alpinin, resin.

Actions: circulatory stimulant, diaphoretic; digestive tonic and carminative.

Applications: to many digestive upsets, particularly flatulence, nausea and vomiting, digestive sluggishness, particularly applied to the effects of cold and a possible remedy in fever management; travel sickness.

Dosage: 0.5-2 grams of dried rhizome equivalent three times per day.

Galega officinalis, goat's rue.

Galium aparine, cleavers.

gall-bladder disease, infection, inflammation, or stone-formation in the muscular sac connected with the bile system draining the liver, responsible for concentrating and storing bile between meals. Gallstones are formed from excessive concentration of bile factors, especially cholesterol; they may be quite symptomless, but under certain conditions can cause severe colic, especially if they move into the bile duct; if the bile duct is blocked a sudden **jaundice** may ensue; inflammation or infection of the gall-bladder (cholecystitis) usually accompanies gallstones, either as a precondition, or as a result of irritation by the stones; it may also occur on its own. Symptoms are pain, typically starting dull and over the stomach, moving out to the right side under the ribs and becoming sharper as the outer wall of the gall-bladder is affected. There is usually a congestive **dyspepsia** and/or heartburn, especially associated with fatty foods. Herbal treatment of all gall-bladder problems centres on remedies that dilute and increase bile flow, i.e., **cholagogues** or the **bitter** digestive stimulants. Other precautions are the same as for **liver disease**. Echinacea is an excellent addition where there is infection. It is exceedingly unlikely that fully-formed gallstones can be broken up or dissolved, although they may be flushed out through the system (combining bitter herbs with lemon juice and olive oil for short periods has a particular reputation for doing this); the possible danger in moving stones is that large ones may become impacted in the bile duct with severe consequences. There is no reason however why gall-bladder inflammation or infection, or even uncalcified stones, may not be relieved.

---

garlic, *Allium sativum* L. Fam: Liliaceae.

The corms or 'cloves' of the familiar culinary article. The fresh cloves are generally the most effective, although the deodorized 'perles' available retain at least some activity.

Habitat: a native of central Asia, but grown in all warm climates, especially southern Europe.

Constituents: volatile oil (containing alliin — this interacts with an enzyme on crushing to convert to allicin, and finally the odorous diallyl disulphide); glucokinins; several minerals including germanium.

Action: anti-pathogenic, particularly in the digestive tract where evidence points to a selective effect against pathogenic colonizations sparing beneficial flora, and also, on account of the antiseptic volatile oil being largely excreted through the body via the lungs, on brochial and pulmonary infections; hypocholesterolaemic and hypolipidaemic; reduces blood-platelet clumping; vasodilatory; expectorant; anti-histaminic.

Applications: to all manner of infections, either as a local application, mouthwash or douche, or internally, where it is particularly effective for infections in the lungs and the gut; notably effective for bronchial conditions; as a long-term treatment for cardiovascular problems, especially atherosclerosis, high blood cholesterol or fat levels, and a predisposition to thrombosis; transiently lowers blood-pressure and probably has a longer benefit as well; a 'warming' remedy very useful for counteracting colds and chills; a notable reputation for healing wounds and reducing the pain and inflammation of stings, etc.; in an oil for earaches and congested middle ear problems; as a digestive aid and a stabilizer of blood sugar levels.

Dosage: 1 clove of raw garlic chopped per day, up to 4-6 for intensive use for short (socially-free!) periods; for long-term treatment 3-6 'perles' per day will be sufficient.

---

gastritis, inflammation or infection of the stomach. May be acute and self-limiting, or chronic. For the former see **dyspepsia;** in the latter case symptoms are lack of appetite, nausea, low-grade vomiting, especially in the morning. These may however be confused with, or lead on to, **ulcers,** or even **cancer,** and should be positively checked. Treatment of gastritis should emphasize improvements in the diet, with strong restrictions on alcohol, smoking and caffeine, and plenty of fruit and vegetables (although some may cause upset). Remedies like Iceland moss, marigold, gum myrrh, comfrey, thyme, Oregon grape, golden seal, cinnamon and licorice may be used as required.

Gaultheria procumbens, wintergreen.

---

gelsemium, Yellow Jasmine root, Wild woodbine, *Gelsemium sempervirens* (L) Ait. Fam: Loganiaceae.

The rhizome and root of a climbing plant with woody, twining stem ascending to very great height on some support trees; leaves are opposite, shining and lanceolate, with, in axillary clusters, large, scented funnel-shaped yellow flowers; the rhizomes (actually underground sections of stem) occur in cylindrical pieces of varying size with stem scars above and roots attached below; the taste is bitter, the odour faintly aromatic.

Habitat: eastern U.S.A. and Central America in moist woodlands and along sea coasts.

Constituents: indole alkaloids (including gelsemine, sempervirine, etc.); gelsemic acid (methyl aesculetin); monomethyl ester of emodin.

Actions: sedative and analgesic; vasodilator and diaphoretic.

Applications: to nerve pains, migraine, toothache; where a strong sedative is needed.

Dosage: maximum permitted dosage is 0.025 gram (25mg) of the dried rhizome and root equivalent three times per day.

Caution: this remedy is very toxic in high doses; it is not permitted to be sold in the U.K. to other than professional practitioners; toxic effects include double vision, lack of balance, and drooping of the eyelids; in larger doses it gives rise to convulsions and death.

Gelsemium sempervirens, gelsemium.

---

gentian, Yellow Gentian, *Gentiana lutea* L. Fam: Gentianaceae.

The rhizome and roots of a perennial herb with a smooth straight stem up to 120cm in height giving off opposite bluish-green elliptical leaves with prominent curved veins; 3-10 yellow flowers arise together in the axils of bowl-shaped bracts; obtained commercially as cylindrical pieces or longitudinally wrinkled, the rhizome often branched and ending in a stem scar; the whole flexible and spongy with a very bitter taste.

Habitat: alpine and sub-alpine pastures of central and southern Europe.

Constituents: bitter glycosides (including gentiopicrin, amaropicrin, amarogentin and amaroswerin); alkaloids (including gentianine); flavonoids (including gentisin).

Actions: pronounced bitter digestive stimulant; anti-inflammatory.

Applications: to digestive atony of any sort, having a beneficial action in even the most sensitive individual; particularly for any anorexia, insufficient digestive secretions, intestinal and gastric inflammations, hepatic and gall-bladder disease; as an adjunct to fever management and in conditions of chronic inflammatory disease where digestion appears to be less than ideal.

Dosage: 0.5-2 grams of dried rhizome and roots three times per day.

Gentiana lutea, Gentian.

---

geranium, *see* **cranesbill, American.**

Geranium maculatum, cranesbill, American.

---

germander, wall, Germander, *Teucrium chamaedrys* L. Fam: Labiatae.

A perennial, almost woody plant, with single stems up to 20cm high; ovate deeply toothed hairy leaves with wedge-shaped base; reddish-purple flowers in whorls of 2-6 of characteristic labiate shape.

Habitat: on banks and walls over Europe, Asia and locally in Britain.

Constituents: bitter principles, flavonoids, tannins, volatile oil.

Actions: gentle bitter and astringent; anti-inflammatory; easing congestive catarrh.

Applications: to debilitated digestion and loss of appetite; diarrhoea in children; for catarrhal conditions of the respiratory system; as a possible constituent of prescriptions for arthritic disease.

Dosage: 1-4 grams of dried herb equivalent three times per day.

Geum urbanum,   avens.

---

ginger, *Zingiber officinale* Rosc. Fam: Zingiberaceae.

The tuberous rhizome familiar in kitchen as a spice and flavouring, available in the dried and powdered form, but for medicinal purposes best in the fresh form.

Habitat: a native of hot climates in Asia and cultivated extensively in the West Indies, Africa and India.

Constituents: volatile oil (including cineole, borneol, linalool, zingiberol, camphene, citral, phellandrene); phenols (gingeol, zingerone); shagaol; and a possible alkaloid.

Actions: a strong circulatory stimulant and vasodilator; diaphoretic; expectorant and pulmonary antiseptic; visceral antispasmodic and carminative.

Applications: as a most comforting and effective remedy for conditions of cold and chill, particularly affecting the lungs and respiratory system; acting like a somewhat more gentle **cayenne** to improve circulation through the tissues and promoting a cleansing diaphoresis; for flatulence and colic.

Dosage: 250-1000mg dried root equivalent (double for fresh) three times a day.

---

ginseng, American, Five-fingers, *Panax quinquefolium* L. Fam: Araliaceae.

The root of a perennial plant with branched rootstock giving rise to a single, slender, smooth stem crowned with a spray of leaves each formed of five separate leaflets with serrated margins, and a single umbel of small yellow flowers giving way in turn to a cluster of red berries; the root is spindle-shaped, 2.5-4cm long and around 1cm across, pale-coloured and mealy in cross-section; it is forked and divided into smaller branches with longitudinal wrinkles; the taste is sweet and mucilaginous.

Habitat: rich woodland through eastern North America; now very rare in the wild and cultivated in a number of locations.

Constituents: triterpenoid saponins (especially ginsenoside Rb and Re).

Actions: mild **adaptogen,** with predominantly relaxing effect specifically effective on the digestive system.

Applications: dyspeptic and anorexic conditions, nausea and vomiting associated with nervous tension or exhaustion.

Dosage: 0.5-4 grams of dried root equivalent three times per day.

---

ginseng, Asiatic, *Panax ginseng* C.A. Meyer. Fam: Araliaceae.

The root of a perennial plant, obtainable in the West as straw-yellow pieces (although there is a red form, the result of a curing process), fleshy but firm, longitudinally wrinkled with root scars, topped by a neck and short rhizome (giving the oldest specimens a sometimes almost human appearance); there is a short fracture and on the internal surface there is a pronounced brown cambium line on the straw-yellow surface; the taste should be clean, slightly sweet at first, then a little bitter. There are many substitutes and inferior samples sold: buying from an accredited graded stock is safest.

Habitat: in the mountainous forests of the northern temperate zone of the Far East, now all but extinct in the wild; grown commercially in Korea, China and elsewhere.

Constituents: triterpenoid saponins (especially ginsenoside Rb and Rg); panax acid; glycosides (panaxin, panaquilin, ginsenin); sterols; essential oil.

Actions: improving the responses of the adrenal cortex in secreting the stress hormones possibly by interacting with receptor sites at the cortex and at the hypothalamus; variously stimulating and relaxing the central nervous system; affecting hepatic metabolism and glycogen utilization by skeletal muscle (to improve muscular stamina without making excessive demands on carbohydrate stores); cardiotonic; hypoglycaemic. In general manifesting in a notable way the **adaptogenic** principle: tending to improve the balance of functions.

Applications: to debilitated, degenerative conditions and the problems of old age; in the *short term* for the improvement of stamina, concentration, healing, stress resistance, vigilance and work efficiency, and the support of the constitution when under attack by stressors.

Dosage: (for the elderly or for the long-term treatment of debilitated conditions): 400-800mg of dried root equivalent per 24 hours. (For the short-term application to stressful conditions in the young): 600-2000mg of dried root equivalent per 24 hours for up to three weeks in any month.

Caution: to be avoided for those reacting to stresses with increased nervous tension or anxiety (e.g., for children and the hyperactive), in women with menstrual irregularities, and along with caffeine. Not to be taken for more than three weeks by the young and active.

---

ginseng, Siberian, Touch-me-not, Devil's Bush, Eleuthero, *Eleutherococcus senticosus* Maxim. Fam: Araliaceae.

The root of a tall bush related to, and with similar foliage to, the Asiatic ginseng, available commercially in proprietary formulations.

Habitat: southern regions of the Soviet Far East, Korea and China.

Constituents: triterpenoid saponins (eleutherosides A-F).

Actions: stimulating **adaptogen**; circulatory stimulant and vasodilator; in substantial ways similar in pharmacology to Asiatic ginseng but probably more stimulating overall.

Applications: to improving stamina in the face of excessive physical and mental demands or exertion; to improving vitality in exhaustion, debility and depression; improving ability to withstand stresses in a general way (e.g., increasing resistance to disease, infections, aging, and especially cold); a claimed effect reversing atherosclerosis (at least in early stages) and a broad range of cardiovascular disturbances, as well as mild to moderate cases of diabetes mellitus. (*Note:* all actions and applications arising out of research in the U.S.S.R; little corroborative investigation has occurred elsewhere.)

Dosage: 0.2-1 gram of dried root equivalent three times a day for up to a month.

Caution: the limitations to the usage of Asiatic ginseng apply at least as much to this remedy: it is even more stimulating in action.

---

glandular fever, an infectious viral disease giving fever, swollen lymphatic glands, with variable course, but typically lasting some weeks and followed by extensive periods of weakness; it is this characteristic which is seized on by herbal practitioners: the condition most often occurs in adolescents and those passing through growing spurts, emotional stress, and in other ways at a low ebb: the disease itself usually heralds a further lowering in reserves and unless properly treated with supportive regimes can lead to many years of reduced defences and liability to other illness. Thus **fever management** is augmented by **nervous restorative** and **anti-infective** remedies, as well as **lymphatic** herbs. As soon as appropriate a concerted campaign of **convalescence** must be instituted, and maintained more or less for weeks or even months if necessary. Only when the patient's return to robustness is unquestioned are such precautions unnecessary.

Glechoma hederacea,   ground ivy.

Glycyrrhiza glabra,   licorice.

Gnaphalium uliginosum,   cudweed, marsh.

---

goat's rue,   French lilac, *Galega officinalis* L. Fam: Papilionaceae.

A handsome perennial herb, about 90-120cm in height, with bushy growth; the masses of largely unbranched stems bear alternate pinnate leaves, each with up to seventeen lanceolate leaflets ending in a small spine; the flowers appear in spikes growing from the leaf axils and are pale blue, lilac or white and papilionate in structure; these give way to long, erect, bean-like seed pods.

Habitat: native to southern Europe and western Asia and found occasionally in Britain as a garden escape; a distinctive contribution to the herbaceous border.

Constituents: alkaloids (including galegine), saponins, bitter principles, tannin, flavonoids.

Actions: galegine is a hypoglycaemic agent and this appears to be the principle action of the whole plant, though direct action at the beta-cells of the pancreas seems to be supplemented here by an influence on protein and lipid metabolism; galactogogue.

Applications: as a component of the management and possible control of late-onset diabetes mellitus (but note caution here) and associated acidosis; to improving milk-flow in lactation.

Dosage: 1-2 grams of dried herb equivalent three times a day (but with close monitoring of blood glucose levels in the early stages of diabetic application).

---

goitre,   *see* **thyroid disease.**

---

golden rod,   *Solidago virgaurea* L. Fam: Compositae.
An upright perennial herb with tufts of stiff stems up to 60cm high bearing numerous radiate yellow flowerheads in crowded, narrow terminal panicles; the leaves are ovate and stalked at the base, narrower up the stem, and slightly toothed.
Habitat: common to woodland throughout Britain, Europe, Asia and North America.
Constituents: saponins, flavonoids, tannins, bitter principle, essential oil, polyacetylenes.
Actions: anti-inflammatory; relaxant; anti-catarrhal; urinary antiseptic.
Applications: to chronic upper respiratory catarrh, urinary infections; flatulent dyspepsia; any of the above cases especially where associated with nervous tension and restlessness.
Dosage: 0.5-2 grams of dried herb equivalent three times per day.

---

golden seal,   Yellow root, Orange root, *Hydrastis canadensis* L. Fam: Ranunculaceae.
The rhizome and roots of a small perennial plant with a single hairy stem producing two five-lobed serrated leaves and a small single apetalous flower with greenish sepals, giving way to a raspberry-like fruit; the rhizome is a bright yellow-brown in colour, twisted and wrinkled with many fine rootlets attached, that breaks easily showing a dark yellow interior; the taste is bitter.
Habitat: rich shady woodlands through north and north-eastern North America, but rare in the wild and usually cultivated for commerce.
Constituents: alkaloids (including berberine, hydrastine and canadine); volatile oil; resin.
Actions: astringent and healing to the gut wall and other mucous membranes; digestive stimulant and cholagogue; laxative; a stimulating adjunct to other remedies for the lungs, kidneys and reproductive tract.
Applications: to states of depressed digestion associated with liver disorder or sensitivity (e.g., to fatty foods and/or alcohol); to gastric and enteric inflammations (e.g., gastritis, enteritis, peptic ulceration) and to excessive gastric sensitivities to food; locally as a mouthwash for gum and mouth disease, as an external application to broken skin and eruptions, as a douche for vaginal problems, as eardrops for middle-ear inflammation and congestion, and as a snuff for nasal inflammation.
Caution: best avoided in pregnancy and in cases of high blood-pressure.

Dosage: 0.5-2 grams of dried rhizome and roots equivalent three times per day.

Gossypium herbaceum et spp,   cotton root.

---

gotu kola,   Hydrocotle, Indian Pennywort, *Centella asiatica* (L) Urban., *Hydrocotyle asiatica* L. Fam: Umbelliferae.

A small umbelliferous herb; kidney-shaped leaves with crenated margin up to 2cm across by 1cm in length, with long narrow petioles.

Habitat: throughout the tropical Near and Far East, particularly in India, Pakistan, Sri Lanka, Madagascar, growing in damp areas above 600 metres above sea-level.

Constituents: an ester, triterpenoid glycosides (including asiaticoside), vallerin, a bitter principle, tannins, alkaloid, volatile oil, pectin.

Actions: restorative and relaxant for the nervous system; bitter digestive stimulant, diuretic and alterative, the whole acting to reduce inflammation and fever; damages the coating of the leprosy bacillus; locally healing and cleansing.

Applications: to neurological and mental disturbances; rheumatic and other inflammatory diseases (such as skin disease); locally for poorly healing wounds, skin inflammations and ulcers. Has an extremely high reputation in India as an **adaptogenic** tonic, and as a treatment for leprous sores and ulcers (modern investigations support this).

Dosage: 0.5-2 grams of dried herb equivalent three times a day for up to a month.

---

gout,   or podogra, is an acutely painful inflammatory disease of the joints brought about by the accummulation of uric acid crystals in the tissues; the affected joint is generally swollen and red and unbearably sensitive to touch and there are often feverish episodes; triggered or exacerbated by rich food, alcohol; generally an inherited predisposition; treatment should commence with a low-purine diet (one that reduces the tendency for the body to produce uric acid), i.e., cutting out fatty fish like mackerel, herring, sardines, etc., shellfish, meat stock, offal, and reducing all meat; attention should also be paid to general principles for an arthritic diet (*see* **arthritis**), and alcohol, caffeine and smoking should be cut out; among the herbs, celery seed specifically increases the elimination of uric acid from the body; other possibilities include heather flowers, devil's claw, birch and asparagus. Other remedies used for arthritis may be appropriate, with particular emphasis on the **diuretics** and **anti-inflammatory** herbs.

---

gravel,   *see* **urinary stones.**

---

gravel root,   Joe-pye weed, Queen-of-the-meadow, Purple boneset, Kidney root, *Eupatorium purpureum* L. Fam: Compositae.

The rhizome and roots of a tall erect perennial herb, up to 3 metres high (but usually 1.5-2),with a hollow stem and whorls of five pointed oblong leaves with roughly-toothed margins, and terminating in heads of purple flowers; the rhizome is hard and fibrous, brown and wrinkled externally, white internally; with bitter and astringent taste.

Habitat: in wet ground in southern Canada and eastern U.S.A.

Constituents: flavonoid (eupatorin), volatile oil, resin.

Actions: diuretic with a soothing effect on the urinary system; tones the pelvic viscera in general.

Applications: to urinary calculi and to soothe urinary infections and irritations; to prostatic inflammation; to spasmodic dysmenorrhoea with scanty menstruation.

Dosage: 1-4 grams of dried rhizome and roots three times per day.

---

grindelia,   Gumplant, Tarweed, *Grindelia camporum* Greene., *et spp.* Fam: Compositae.

Biennial or perennial herbs and shrubs with smooth stems giving rise to alternate light-green, coarsely toothed leaves with a clasping base, and terminating in single large yellow flowerheads; they are covered, when young, in a sticky varnish.

Habitat: coastal areas of western North America.

Constituents: saponins (including grindelin), volatile oil, bitter alkaloid (grindeline), resin, tannins.

Actions: relaxing expectorant and antispasmodic; bradycardic action on the heart.

Applications: to bronchial spasm in asthma, asthmatic bronchitis, and nervous, irritable and dry cough; when above conditions are associated with tachycardia.

Dosage: 1-3 grams of dried herb equivalent three times per day.

Caution: large doses of this remedy may irritate the kidneys.

Grindelia camporum et spp,   grindelia.

---

ground ivy, Alehoof, Creeping Jenny, *Nepeta hederacea* (L) Trev., *Glechoma hederacea* L. Fam: Labiatae.

A creeping perennial herb with more or less hairy long-stalked, crenated, ovate-cordate leaves arising from extensive rooting stems; flowering stems arise up to 30cm high with large blue labiate flowers in groups of six in axillary whorls; in bright sun the leaves become red or purple.

Habitat: common invasive weed in gardens and waste places, preferring heavier soil, throughout the temperate northern hemisphere.

Constituents: bitter principle (glechomine), tannins, volatile oil.

Actions: astringent, anticatarrhal.

Applications: to upper respiratory catarrhal problems, including middle ear infections and sinus congestion; used as a mouthwash and gargle for local inflammations of the mouth and throat; for chronic bronchial catarrh; as an astringent remedy for inflammations in the digestive tract and haemorrhoids.

Dosage: 1-4 grams of the dried herb equivalent three times per day.

Guaiacum officinale et spp, lignum vitae.

---

gum disease, whether inflammation, gingivitis, or the more serious purulent form, pyorrhoea, is caused primarily by bacterial plaque and eating refined and sugary foods. The elimination of these is thus a high priority, and hopes for effective treatment must be very low unless this is done. It may also be that the gums have broken down to the extent that pockets form between the upper gums and the teeth and these will need dental surgery, gingivectomy. It is however possible to improve and maintain gum health with mouthwashes made up with thyme, myrrh, marigold, sage, blackberry leaf, rhatany, wild indigo or tormentil, preferably in tincture form. Gum disease may proceed to periodontal problems where the tooth roots are loosened and inflammation or infection spreads deep into the jaw. Mouthwashes and other measures are still applicable to treat the gums, but internal **anti-infective** and **alterative** treatment will also be necessary.

H

haemorrhoids, varicosed veins of the rectum leading to their swelling and often bleeding when emptying the bowels; by far the most common cause of bleeding at stool, but should be confirmed by qualified practitioner. Possibly precipitated by straining when moving the bowels (i.e., by constipation), lack of exercise, pregnancy, or inherent weakness of the veins (*see* **varicose veins**). Priority in treatment should be to ease bowel movements with **aperients**, dietary fibre and exercise. Direct treatment for the haemorrhoids internally is the same as for varicose veins; externally, in the form of a gel or paste, such remedies as witch hazel, pilewort, tormentil root, comfrey, rhatany, or any **astringent** herb, will be most useful.

---

haemostatic, a term used for a remedy that can check bleeding; this can be achieved locally by most herbs of the **astringent** group; where bleeding is from the lungs, urinary system, rectum or other internal aperture, then qualified practitioners should be consulted to assess the causes, as these may occasionally be serious.

Hamamelis virginiana, witch hazel.

Harpagophytum procumbens, devil's claw.

Hart's tongue fern, *Phyllitis scolopendrium* (L) Newm., *Scolopendrium vulgare* Sym. Fam: Polypodiaceae.

A fern with undivided glossy-green strap-like leaves, with rows of sori on each side of the midrib on the underside, set at about 60° to it.

Habitat: shady banks, walls and similar locations throughout Britain, Europe, Asia and north-western North America.

Constituents: methylglutamic acid and other amino acids.

Actions: astringent; reputed to clear liver conditions.

Applications: to intestinal irritations and diarrhoea; to splenic enlargement and other signs of portal hypertension.

Dosage: 1-4 grams of dried leaves equivalent three times per day.

---

hawthorn, Mayflower, Whitethorn, Quickset, *Crataegus oxyacanthoides* (*C. monogyna*) L. Fam: Rosaceae.

The flowers, leaves or fruit of a deciduous shrubby tree with smooth thorny shoots and three-lobed stipulate leaves; small white or pink flowers are arranged in corymbs and on long stalks, each with prominent stamens around the nectary and carpels; the haw berry is red with white mealy flesh and a large stone.

Habitat: in hedgerows and copses throughout Britain and all temperate regions of the northern hemisphere.

Constituents: flavonoid glycosides (including rutin and quercitrin), saponins, cyanogenic glycosides, trimethylamine, condensed tannins.

Action: coronary and peripheral vasodilator, also having a bradycardic effect on the myocardium; it appears to exert a tonifying action on the tissues of the vasculature.

Applications: to heart conditions — the twin almost paradoxical effects on the heart, the dilating of the coronary blood supply and the tendency to slow down and stabilize the contractility of the heart muscle mean that it finds many applications to heart disturbances (these must, however, never be treated without professional experience of the issues involved); also applicable to peripheral circulatory conditions, such as intermitent claudication and other problems of atherosclerosis.

Dosage: 0.25-1 gram dried flowers, leaves or fruit equivalent three times a day.

---

hay fever, an allergic rhinitis triggered by inhalation of grass and other pollen, often inherited as an allergic predisposition which may show itself as asthma, allergic eczema, or food allergies as well. May also be acquired or triggered by early exposure in infancy to cow's milk or other 'foreign' foods before the digestive system can render such protein harmless: ongoing allergy to cow's milk or other foods is well worth investigating (*see* **food allergies**). Apart from avoiding pollen or other allergens as far as possible relief may be had by using herbal remedies that tone up the respiratory mucosa, like ribwort, ground ivy, goldenrod, cudweed or golden seal, practitioners often use ma-huang to reduce the aggressiveness of the sensitivity response. Treatment, however, is often most complex.

---

headache, a very common but complex condition that can arise from a great variety of causes; the most common cause is spasm of the blood vessels to the head, but this itself may be due to a range of factors: anxiety and worry, muscle strain throughout the neck, shoulders and scalp, excessive alcohol intake, a feverish illness, **arteriosclerosis, high blood-pressure, hypoglycaemia,** or there may be a clear-cut syndrome: **migraine.** Apart from dealing with the primary problem, it is often possible to help such headaches with remedies that regulate peripheral blood vessels, such as limeflowers, betony, rosemary, the **peripheral vasodilators,** and lavender oil applied externally. Other causes of headaches must be treated at root as far as possible; they include **neuralgia,** eyestrain, glaucoma, **sinusitis,** sunstroke, tooth decay and **kidney disease;** in acute or puzzlingly chronic conditions the possibility of brain haemorrhage, tumour or thrombosis must be considered. These causes apart, most headaches will respond to the use of **relaxants** and/or **antispasmodics;** it will be wise to differentiate 'hot' and 'cold' types before treatment (*see* **migraine**). It is also possible that a condition will be contributed to by sluggish bowels and other poor eliminations and thus **laxatives** and appropriate **eliminative remedies** may be useful: the same approach justifies the use of the **hepatic** herbs in some cases.

healing remedies, herbs that promote healing in wounded or inflamed tissues include in different ways the **demulcent** and **astringent** remedies; particular examples however are comfrey, chickweed and marigold flowers.

heartburn, pain in the region of the heart caused by excessive acidity of the gastric juices; often accompanied by burning sensation up to the back of the throat. A symptom of **hiatus hernia;** *see also* **hyperacidity.**

heart problems, there are a number of herbal remedies that have a useful effect on poor heart function. These range from **cardioactive** remedies like lily-of-the-valley, through ephedra and broom, to the more supportive **cardiotonic** remedies such as hawthorn, motherwort, rosemary and mistletoe. These remedies allow the herbal practitioner to help in many heart conditions such as heart failure, **arrythmia,** and coronary heart disease and **angina pectoris;** however, many sufferers are already taking conventional heart drugs and this may inhibit safe treatment with herbs: for this reason and because heart disease has its own obvious dangers, it is strongly recommended that unqualified people do not attempt treatment.

heartsease, Pansy, Herb trinity, *Viola tricolor* L. Fam: Violaceae.
An annual or perennial herb up to 40cm in height with branching stems,

either erect or creeping, bearing small opposite elongated oval leaves with crenated margins, and with divided leaflets at the base of each stalk; the flowers are characteristically three-coloured, purple, yellow and white: the upper two petals paired and purple, the bottom of the five being broad and with yellow at the base.

Habitat: hilly pastures and banks, invading waste places and fallow ground, throughout Britain, Europe and Asia.

Constituents: saponins, salicylates, alkaloid, flavonoids, tannin, mucilage.

Actions: expectorant; anti-inflammatory; laxative; diuretic.

Applications: skin conditions, especially discharging eczema; rheumatic conditions and bronchial infections; at its best in complex syndromes such as auto-immune disease where several of these conditions are combined.

Dosage: 1-4 grams of dried herb equivalent three times per day.

---

heather flowers, Ling flowers, *Calluna vulgaris* L. Fam: Ericaceae.

The pale pink or white flowers of a straggling shrub up to 100cm high with very short overlapping leaves prolonged below their base, either hairy or very smooth.

Habitat: very widely distributed in acid soils over Britain, central and northern Europe, rarely in North America.

Constituents: alkaloid (ericodin), arbutin, tannin, flavonoids.

Actions: diuretic and urinary antiseptic.

Applications: to urinary infections such as cystitis and urethritis; gouty and other arthritic conditions.

Dosage: 1-2 grams of the dried foliage equivalent three times per day.

Helonias dioica et spp, helonias root.

---

helonias root, False unicorn root, Devil's bit, *Chamaelirium luteum* (L.) Gray., *Helonias dioica* (Pursh.), *H. lutea* (Ker-Gawl)., *C. carolianum* (Wild)., *Veratrum luteum* L. Fam: Liliaceae.

The rhizome of a herbaceous perennial about 30-100cm in height, with smooth angular stems, alternate spatulate to lanceolate leaves, with numerous small greenish-white flowers arranged in a dense terminal raceme; the rhizome is bulbous, grey-brown outside, closely annulated, with a horn-coloured smooth interior.

Habitat: a native of low, moist ground in the Mississippi area of the U.S.A.

Constituents: steroidal saponins (including chamaelirin).

Actions: improving the secretory responses and cyclical functions of the ovary, appearing to have an **adaptogenic** effect on this organ.

Applications: to menstrual irregularities, particularly those of menstruation itself and the first half of the cycle (up to ovulation); to infertility caused by dysfunction in follicular formation; to functional ovarian cysts and to aid in resolving other ovarian pathologies; to salpingo-oophoritis; to threatened miscarriages.

Dosage: 1-2 grams of dried rhizome equivalent three times per day.

---

henbane, Hogbean, *Hyoscyamus niger* L. Fam: Solanaceae.

A coarse, erect, branching annual up to 60cm high with large sessile, irregularly-divided, hairy leaves; the dull yellow flowers have prominent purple veins and arise closely from branches or forks; the globular seed capsule contains numerous small seeds; the whole plant has a nauseous odour.

Habitat: on rough and waste ground scattered throughout Britain, Europe and northern North America, and more commonly through southern Europe and western Asia.

Constituents: alkaloids (including hyoscyamine, hyoscine and scopalamine).

Actions: antispasmodic on smooth muscle; sedative; anticholinergic.

Applications: to bronchial spasm in asthma and whooping cough; to prevent colic and griping in the gut and urinary system; reducing tremor and spasm generally; preventing travel sickness.

Dosage: restricted to a maximum of 100mg of the dried herb equivalent three times per day: recommended dose is no more than 30mg.

Caution: this is a dangerous remedy in untrained hands; under the terms of the Medicines Act 1968 its use is confined to professional medical herbalists; the same precautions and risks attend its use as they do deadly nightshade, to which reference must be made.

---

hepatic, a term used for a remedy that enhances liver function; herbalists have traditionally been particularly attentive to liver function (dealing as they used to with many cases of jaundice, and recalling the very ancient associations that the liver had with life, soul and emotions), and this is reflected in the character of many remedies, which often have some effect in this area. Most such remedies are **cholagogues,** but there are others less dynamic that can in their different ways be seen as nurturing or toning the liver in its many metabolic, detoxifying, regulatory and even immunological-control activities; they are indicated whenever clinical examination provides clues that the liver is particularly under assault or is not functioning well. Examples are dandelion root, milk thistle, artichoke, centaury, black root, Hart's-tongue and bittersweet.

---

hepatitis, infection and/or inflammation of the liver, due to infective or toxic factors, occurring in a wide variety of forms; the condition may be acute or chronic, and can vary from the mildly transient to the very severe. The most common infective types are viral, hepatitis A generally being transmitted by faecal-oral contamination, hepatitis B mostly (but not always) by direct contamination of the bloodstream. The former is generally far less severe and lasting than the latter, and is particularly associated with poor hygiene, diet, crowded conditions, and is most common in the young. Hepatitis B is notably spread by contaminated needles and other items that puncture the skin, but in fact in most cases arises from no such apparent event: it is particularly likely to lead on to chronic or chronic-active hepatitis. Other infective organisms can cause hepatitis; it may also arise from industrial and other chemical poisons, or may proceed from internal immunological disorders. In all but the simplest cases therefore it is a most complex condition. Symptoms are variable, but include nausea and vomiting, diarrhoea, lack of appetite, fever and jaundice; the stools and urine may be darker or paler. The intricacies of hepatitis are such that only qualified practitioners should be entrusted with its care, and doctors should also be consulted for laboratory and other examinations (this especially so for contagious forms). In general, however, strict hygiene must be observed, the diet must be very light and simple and especially free of fats and alcohol. Smoking should also stop. It is unwise to launch into a specific herbal regime without understanding the nature of the condition, as it is quite likely that the condition will be exacerbated. In practice, gentle **hepatic** remedies like dandelion root, milk thistle seed and artichoke provide the best foundations for treatment; any fever will have to be managed conservatively with appropriate remedies, as will excessive diarrhoea or vomiting. **Cholagogues** and strong **bitters** should only be used when it is expertly judged wise to do so. Background factors will, as always, demand treatment. It is often necessary to continue following up liver treatment a long time after the disease has passed, *see* **liver disease**.

---

herbalism, any system of medicine or health-care that relies on plants as the source of remedies; as seen principally: (1) in almost all cultures prior to the impact of the Industrial Revolution, mostly as a self-help therapy but exemplified in the hands of locally-trained rural practitioners (*see* **traditional medicine**); and (2) as a substantial modern alternative to conventional drug-based medicine (*see* **medical herbalism, phytotherapy**). In most countries traditional and modern usages coexist; thus herbalism today is based on remedies and techniques tried and tested through generations of use, but increasingly re-evaluated in the light of modern medical refinements. A key feature of herbalism is that remedies are used to support and modify disturbed body functions, rather than to directly attack the symptoms of disease.

---

herpes, in fact herpes simplex, to distinguish it from herpes zoster (*see* **shingles**), a viral infection that typically produces 'cold sores' around the mouth, and small blisters that, when ruptured leave a thin yellowish crust, often exacerbated by broken skin or fissures, and very prone to secondary infection. The same virus is responsible for the sexually-transmitted or venereal herpes, where the blisters break out on the genitalia. Predisposing or triggering factors responsible for break-outs include local irritation or trauma, sunlight, hormonal disturbances such as occur in menstruation, pregnancy or emotional trauma, other infections, and beyond that any general lowering of resistance. Attention to any of these and treatment with hormonal **adaptogens, nervous restoratives, anti-infective, relaxant** and **eliminative** remedies are quite likely to contain, if not dispel, the problem.

---

hiatus hernia, a protrusion of the stomach upwards through the diaphragm, at the point through which the oesophagus opens into it. Mostly after periods of raised intra-abdominal pressure such as chronic constipation (often associated with this and gall-bladder disease simultaneously — 'Saint's Triad'), pregnancy, obesity and a long period of heavy lifting. Marked by heartburn and reflux into the mouth especially on stooping and lying down, dyspepsia and other discomforts. Any damage is not treatable except by surgical means, but relief from the symptoms may be had by reducing constipation and obesity, and using soothing mucilages like slippery elm before and after meals. Excess stomach acid may be controlled as well, *see* **hyperacidity**.

Hieracium pilosella, mouse-ear.

---

high blood-pressure, or hypertension, is a usually quiet condition of raised hydraulic pressure in the circulation; its cause is, in most cases, unknown, but the health of the kidneys is central, as are any hardening of the arteries **(arteriosclerosis)**, hormonal mechanisms, and long-term stress. Treatment of the condition starts out as for arteriosclerosis, with the added dietary advice to reduce salt intake, and with such specific herbal remedies as hawthorn, limeflowers, buckwheat, yarrow and **diuretics** and **relaxants** as appropriate. Quite substantial falls in blood pressure are seen with careful herbal treatment.

---

hops, *Humulus lupulus* L. Fam: Cannabinaceae.

The female 'strobiles' of a perennial climbing plant with annual stems running up to 6 metres in height, giving rise to large 3-5 lobed sharply-toothed leaves with very rough surface; the flowers are single-sexed: the male in loose panicles in the upper leaf axils; the female in closely-stacked cone-like catkins made up of bracts with tiny flowers tucked into the bract axils; after fertilization the cones grow threefold up to 5cm in length and change from pale greenish-yellow to yellow-brown: these are the strobiles of commerce; their smell is heavy and their taste bitter.

Habitat: through Europe to Asia and southern England in hedgerows, thickets and open woods; wild plants and escapes from cultivation are equally encountered.

Constituents: volatile oil and bitter-resin complex (together referred to as 'lupulin'), condensed tannins, oestrogenic substances, asparagin.

Actions: sedative, visceral antispasmodic, bitter digestive tonic, locally antiseptic and healing.

Applications: to visceral smooth muscle tensions affecting digestive and bowel function (e.g., nervous dyspepsia and colitis, spastic constipation); as a bitter tonic to digestion; as a sedative to encourage restfulness and sleep and reducing symptoms of nervous tension; as an inhalant to induce sleep.

Dosage: 0.5-1 gram of dried strobiles three times per day.

Caution: avoid in depressive illness.

---

horehound, black, *Ballota nigra* L. Fam: Labiatae.

A coarse, erect, hairy, branching perennial up to 90cm high with a pronounced foetid smell and purple labiate flowers in dense axillary clusters accompanied by stiff linear bracts; the leaves are stalked, and coarsely toothed.

Habitat: waysides, hedgerows and waste ground throughout Britain, Europe, northern Asia, and naturalized in the eastern U.S.A.

Constituents: flavonoids, volatile oil.
Actions: anti-emetic; relaxant, especially to the digestive tract.
Applications: to vomiting, especially of pregnancy, but to any other of central, digestive or hypoglycaemic origin; to nervous dyspepsia.
Dosage: 1-4 grams of dried herb equivalent three times per day.

---

horehound, white,   Hoarhound, Horehound, *Marrubium vulgare* L. Fam: Labiatae.
A mint-like plant densely covered in white fur, up to 50cm high with thick stem and wrinkled leaves; dense whorls of off-white flowers are found in the upper leaf axils; there is a pronounced bitter taste.
Habitat: roadsides and waste places throughout central and southern Europe and central and northern Asia; scattered throughout Britain and North America.
Constituents: sesquiterpene bitters (including marrubin), essential oil (including marrubiol), mucilage, tannins.
Actions: gently stimulating expectorant; gentle circulatory stimulant; relaxant and antispasmodic; bitter digestive and hepatic tonic.
Applications: to bronchitis and chesty colds especially in congestive catarrhal conditions with non-productive coughing; to ease whooping cough.
Dosage: 0.5-2 grams of dried herb equivalent three times per day.

---

hormonal remedies,   when hormonal disturbances are an important feature of a problem, the herbal approach is to try and understand what underlying destabilizing factors are present rather than simply prescribing substitute hormones; the interpretation is best left to a qualified practitioner, who will often treat the patient in ways quite separate from that apparently indicated by the hormonal disturbance. There are however particular remedies that appear to enhance endocrine functions, often so as to help resolve contradictory hormonal problems equally well (*see* **adaptogen**). These include the ginseng group, helonias root, agnus-castus and saw palmetto; other hormonally active remedies include cotton root, wild yam, damiana, sarsaparilla, licorice, kelp, squaw vine and blue cohosh (*see also* **saponins**).

---

horseradish,   *Armoracia rusticana* (Gaertn.) Mey & Scherb. *Cochlearia armoracia* L. Fam: Cruciferae.
The root of a plant notable for its large (30-50cm) shiny, deep-green

lanceolate toothed leaves (with some pinnate variations) and flowering stems ending in a bunch of small four-petalled white flowers. The fresh root is white and marked by the characteristic pungent aroma and burning taste.

Habitat: introduced for cultivation from eastern Europe, now widespread along field boundaries, waste places and waysides favouring slightly damp and shady positions, throughout Britain and Europe.

Constituents: mustard oil glycosides (including sinigrin), ascorbic acid, asparagin, resin.

Actions: strong circulatory stimulant; antiseptic action, notably for lungs and urinary system, when taken internally (due to excretion of mustard oils at these sites); diuretic; promoting healing; stimulating stomach secretions.

Applications: like **cayenne** as a central constituent of prescriptions applied to conditions marked by poor circulation or cold; externally to stimulate circulation over inflamed joints or tissues; for pulmonary and urinary infections and for urinary stones and oedematous conditions; to help eliminate infections and infestations of the upper digestion.

Dosage: 2-4 grams of fresh root taken three times per day before meals.

Caution: like all members of the cabbage and mustard family horseradish tends to depress thyroid function: it should be avoided where thyroid levels are low.

---

horsetail, Shavegrass, Pewterwort, Bottlebrush, *Equisetum arvense* L. Fam: Equisetaceae.

The sterile growth of this member of a very primitive family of plants that once covered the planet (and formed much of our coal deposits); in spring a spore-bearing stem, resembling a thin asparagus shoot, rises 15-20cm; once shed, this is replaced by a pale-green bush with erect hollow jointed stems with longitudinal furrows, and with sharply-toothed sheaths covering each joint; from the sheaths of the central stem arise whorls of fine branches, each giving off further whorls, the whole extending up to 60cm in height.

Habitat: in moist waste places throughout temperate regions of the world.

Constituents: silica (up to 10 per cent), saponin, alkaloids (including nicotine and palustrene), bitter principle, flavonoids, many minerals in abundance.

Actions: astringent and styptic effect on the urinary mucosa; strong diuretic; restorative to damaged pulmonary tissue; supporting the inflammatory response; possible detoxifier.

Applications: to urinary and prostatic disease for the relief of symptoms and possibly to help in healing (its ability to promote leucocytosis is suggested as accounting for its ability to help in prostatic and urinary inflammations); to contribute to managing enuresis and other irritable symptoms of the urinary system; to the repair of lung damage after pulmonary tuberculosis and other disease; as a diuretic particularly suited to metabolic or hormonal oedema.

Dosage: 1-4 grams of dried herb (by decoction) three times per day.

Caution: often recommended for blood in the urine: always refer this for professional treatment.

---

hot flushes, *see* **menopause.**

'hot' remedies, *see* **circulatory stimulants.**

---

hot spices, *see* **circulatory stimulants.**

Humulus lupulus, hops.

Hydrangea arborescens, seven barks.

Hydrastis canadensis, golden seal.

Hydrocotyle asiatica, gotu kola.

Hyoscyamus niger, henbane.

---

hyperacidity, excessive production of stomach acid and digestive juices, giving acid dyspepsia (indigestion controllable by antacids) and predisposing to gastritis and peptic ulcers. Definitely linked with stress, especially around mealtimes, and made worse by eating hot spices, meat products, and alcohol and coffee. However, many cases persist even without such triggers. Mucilaginous herbs will reduce the symptoms of the excess acid (notably slippery elm, meadowsweet, comfrey, marshmallow, Iceland moss and licorice) and sweet flag may help to reduce the acidity directly. Antacids are *not* a good idea, as they tend to prolong the problem. Treatment of underlying causes is difficult and will differ considerably in different sufferers. **Relaxants,** especially chamomile and lemon balm, will often help.

Hypericum perforatum,   St John's Wort.

---

hypoglycaemia,   low blood sugar; an established condition in only a few, but a functional or 'reactive' form with vacillation of the normally very stable blood sugar levels is very common. Due primarily to stressing of the hormonal pancreas and insulin secretion by excessive consumption of refined carbohydrates, leading to surges of insulin secretion and actual lowering of blood sugar levels shortly after eating; contributory factors are relative exhaustion of the hyperglycaemic stress hormones, and disturbances of serotonin metabolism. Periods of low blood sugar are marked by 'false' hunger soon after eating, and a strong desire for something sweet, especially chocolate; symptoms of irritability, lack of concentration, headache are common and the condition can contribute to many other problems; taking more sweet, merely prolongs the instability of blood sugar control by constantly stressing innate balancing mechanisms. The diet should strictly ban all refined carbohydrates, cocoa and caffeine-containing products, and alcohol in excess, and replace with wholegrains, pulses, vegetables, fruit, etc. Hypoglycaemic crises can be countered effectively by tasting **bitters,** and these should be taken strong as a regular part of the regime: it is hard work.

---

hyssop,   *Hyssopus officinalis* L. Fam: Labiatae.
   A perennial herb of bushy habit with square stems and small narrow leaves, with whorls of blue-violet flowers in the upper axils; the odour and taste of the plant are strong and characteristic.
   Habitat: light dry soil in southern Europe, but widely cultivated elsewhere.
   Constituents: volatile oil, flavonoids, tannin.
   Actions: peripheral vasodilator and diaphoretic; relaxing expectorant; carminative.
   Applications: to coughs and colds and respiratory infections, especially in children, and those of tense or nervous disposition; to help manage influenza attacks.

Dosage: 1-4 grams of dried herb equivalent three times a day.

Hyssopus officinalis, hyssop.

I

Iceland moss, *Cetraria islandica* (L) Ach. Fam: Parmeliaceae.

A lichen with variable uneven thalli, thin and fringed with minute papillae, rarely more than 5mm in width, the whole being quite tough and springy; the undersurface is paler than the upper and covered with depressed white spots; the taste is bitter and mucilaginous.

Habitat: on barren stony ground throughout all northern countries and mountainous areas elsewhere; it is locally common in Britain.

Constituents: mucilages (including lichenin), bitter acids.

Actions: soothing and healing on the gastric wall; nourishing; locally demulcent and healing.

Applications: to gastritis and other irritation and inflammation of the stomach; to contain vomiting arising from such a cause; particularly useful in stomach problems in cachexic and debilitated conditions.

Dosage: 1-2 grams of dried lichen equivalent three times per day.

Ilex paraguariensis, maté.

---

impetigo, highly infectious skin disease found most commonly among school children; marked by blistering on the face leaving discharging lesions with golden crusts. Isolation of the sufferer is essential. Poor hygiene, overcrowding and poor diet are predisposing. Local treatment with antiseptic solution is necessary. Internal treatment with **alteratives,** and remedies to improve digestion, should be combined with a healthy, cleansing diet.

---

impotence, in the man is usually a complex condition, but most often with a psychological or behavioural component; to the extent that this is so, the use of damiana, Asiatic ginseng and saw palmetto are likely to be useful, and the use of appropriate **relaxants** may be indicated. *See also* **infertility.**

---

indigestion, *see* **dyspepsia.**

---

indigo, *see* **wild indigo.**

---

infertility, can arise from a large number of conditions, many of which cannot be identified in any single case; for the woman, ovarian dysfunction can be often corrected with helonias root and agnus-castus, chronic **pelvic inflammation** can often be corrected before permanent obstruction of the fallopian tubes occurs, and general non-specific application of helonias root, blue cohosh and dong quai are all linked with increasing fertility, in some cases dramatically so; for the man, improved fertility is possibly achieved through taking damiana, saw palmetto, oats and sarsaparilla.

---

inflammation, the normal reaction of any body tissue to injury or irritation, characterized for two millennia as occurring in four stages: rubour, calour, dolour and tumour (redness, heat, pain and swelling). These may be explained further as resulting from a histamine-induced dilation of the local small arteries along with the weakening of their walls and the leakage into the surrounding spaces of white blood cells and fluid. The purpose of this activity is to bring to the site of injury as much as possible of the body's defensive capability, particularly white blood cells. Once their job is complete, and the bacteria, virus, toxins or other irritation is dealt with, resolution quickly occurs, although there may be a transient stage when dead white blood cells and bacteria (pus) will need removal, most often by the body's eliminative functions. The herbalist, therefore, does not see inflammation itself as a problem, although it can be painful and disabling. It only becomes a subject of treatment when it cannot cope with the task, i.e., it becomes chronic. Chronic inflammation, is, in one form or other, one of the most common problems of the present day. Arthritis, skin disease, the auto-immune diseases, diverticulitis and chronic bronchitis are only a few of many examples. Whilst modern medicine prescribes anti-inflammatory drugs to suppress the inflammation, the herbalist aims to improve the cleansing of the affected site, side-stepping the inflammation or enhancing its efficiency. Thus **circulatory stimulant and eliminative** remedies are commonly used (on locally accessible sites, such as joints, circulatory stimulation may be most effectively achieved by use of **rubefacients** or even **vesicants**). **Anti-inflammatory** remedies often work to directly enhance or contain the inflammatory processes. Beyond these options the herbalist will always be concerned to reduce the source of toxic, irritant or infective material at source, e.g., from diet, digestive tract, poor liver, kidney or other eliminative functions.

influenza, a common contagious viral infection of the lungs, leading to fever, body pains, coughing, nausea and vomiting, in most cases developing on from what appears to be a common cold. Treatment involves **fever management** remedies and regimes, with especial emphasis on such herbs as elderflowers, garlic, ammoniac, ginger, horseradish, echinacea, pleurisy root and other **expectorant** remedies as appropriate.

infusion, a preparation made by steeping remedies in hot water. Generally lighter material like leaves and flowers is most suitable, though finely ground or powdered root, bark or woody material may be used too (but *see* **decoction**). Most simply, the technique involves adding boiling water to the herb in a container that is then closed as firmly as possible to prevent loss of volatile elements (a vacuum flask is ideal for the purpose). The herb should be steeped for at least 20-30 minutes for optimum extraction. After cooling and straining the liquid may be kept in a refrigerator for several days, but otherwise its keeping qualities are minimal (*see also* **tincture**).

inhalations, medicinal agents carried in a volatile form so as to affect the respiratory mucous membranes; mentholated preparations may be of this form, but the most useful variety is that carried on steam: the herb or preparation is dropped onto the surface of steaming water and the volatile oil/steam mixture is inhaled, often in a makeshift towel 'tent'; the technique is a useful one for relieving nasal congestion, inflammation and hypersensitivity. Herbs with a large **volatile oil** component are most suitable: notable examples are chamomile, eucalyptus, pine, cassia, thyme, rosemary, aniseed, hyssop, lavender and, in moderation, peppermint, and the purified constituents menthol and camphor.

insomnia, a considered approach to this problem will begin with an assessment of all possible contributory factors; provided these are being treated as far as practical, it is then possible to devise a regime of herbal treatment to help sleep to occur at the desired time: this may as much involve **stimulants** and **restoratives** at some times of the day (usually in the morning) as **sedatives** or **relaxants.** The aim throughout is to avoid a state of dependence and an overly depressive effect: thus calming agents should initially be of the gentlest variety, starting with chamomile, limeflowers, vervain or lemon balm, moving through hops, scullcap, valerian, cowslip, or passionflower, to the more sedative lady's slipper, wild lettuce, Jamaican dogwood only if absolutely necessary, and for as short a time as possible; throughout the use of **nervous restoratives** as background will help maintain strength.

---

intermittent claudication, inadequate arterial bloodflow to one or both legs due to **arteriosclerosis,** typically felt as disabling cramp when walking, so that the sufferer has to stop frequently to recover (hence 'shopwindow syndrome'). Treat as for arteriosclerosis , and by graduated leg exercises to improve collateral circulation: specific herbal remedies are prickly ash and hawthorn, but other **peripheral vasodilators** and **circulatory stimulants** may be appropriate. *See also* **Buerger's disease** *and* **Raynaud's disease.**

Inula helenium, elecampane.

---

ipecacuanha, Ipecac, (a) Rio, Matto Grosso, Brazilian or Minas ipecacuanha, *Cephaelis ipecacuanha* (Brot) A. Rich; (b) Cartagena, Costa Rica, Nicaragua or Panama ipecacuanha, *C. acuminata* Karsten. Fam: Rubiaceae.

The root of two species of shrubby plant about 30cm high with partly procumbent or even subterranean stem; the roots are obtained as twisted, tortuous or sometimes beaded brown to red-brown pieces with thick starchy bark and a dense splintering core. Rio ipecacuanha is recognized by its smaller pieces, around 6mm wide as against up to 10mm for the Cartagena, and by the presence of complete annulations around the root at 1-2mm intervals. The taste of both is bitter.

Habitat: moist, shady woods in South and Central America.

Constituents: isoquinoline alkaloids (including emetine, cephaeline, psychotrine); ipecacuanhic acid (a mixture possibly based on a saponin); ipecacuanhin. Rio ipecacuanha, contains much more emetine than cephaeline; in Cartagena the relationship is reversed.

Actions: emetic and stimulating expectorant; peripheral vasodilator and diaphoretic; antiprotozoal.

Applications: to congestive pulmonary conditions such as chronic bronchitis and pertussis; to amoebic dysentery; under certain circumstances and only under trained supervision, as an **emetic.**

Dosage: 25-100mg of dried root equivalent three times per day; the emetic dose is 0.5-2 grams.

Irish moss,   Carragheen, Chondrus, *Chondrus crispus* (L) Stackh. Fam: Gigartinaceae.

A seaweed or red alga, purple to green when fresh but dried to yellow-brown translucent forked fronds or thalli; these are 5-25cm long, almost cylindrical at the base but fanning out in the upper region, and deeply cleft; the odour is slightly seaweed-like, the taste a little salty.

Habitat: the Atlantic coasts of Ireland, Europe and the United States.

Constituents: polysaccharides (carragheen) forming a gel in the presence of potassium ions, protein.

Actions: nutritive and demulcent; relaxing expectorant; emulsifying agent.

Applications: to dyspeptic conditions, with nausea and hyperacidity; as a soothing tonic for convalescence; for irritable cough conditions; as an emulsifying agent with other remedies and applications.

Dosage: 2-10 grams of the dried thallus equivalent three times per day.

Iris versicolor et spp,   blue flag.

---

ispaghula,   *see* **psyllium.**

J

Jamaica dogwood,   Fish poison bark, *Piscidia erythrina* L. Fam: Leguminosae.

The bark of a tree obtained in curved or channelled pieces with grey-brown (or orange-brown if cork is still present) outer surface, and red-brown inner surface, ridged (externally) and furrowed (internally) longitudinally, with a fibrous fracture; the taste is bitter and acrid.

Habitat: West Indies, Florida, Texas, Mexico and northern South America.

Constituents: amorphous alkaloid; glycosides (including piscidin, jamaicin, ichthyone); flavonoids (including sumatrol, rotenone, piscidone, piscerythrone); resin.

Actions: analgesic and sedative.

Applications: neuralgias, toothache, migraine, spasmodic dysmenorrhoea and other pains; insomnia associated with pain or excessive nervous tension.

Dosage: 0.5-2 grams of dried bark equivalent three times per day.

Caution: although not as poisonous to humans as to cold-blooded creatures, this is a remedy to be used with great care, and only by trained practitioners.

---

jambul,   Jamba, Java plum, *Syzygium cumini* L., *Eugenia jambolana* Lamk. Fam: Myrtaceae.

The fruit of a tree up to 10 metres in height, with peach-like leaves, and terminal bunches of greenish-yellow flowers giving way to apricot-like fruit, containing a single brown-black seed; it has a pungent odour and bitter-sweet taste.

Habitat: South-East Asia, India.

Constituents: volatile oil, tannins, resin.

Actions: carminative and astringent; reputed hypoglycaemic.

Applications: to contain and manage diarrhoea, especially when accompanied by colic pains; traditionally used for diabetes mellitus.

Dosage: 0.3-2 grams of dried fruit equivalent three times per day.

Jateorhiza palmata,   calumba.

---

jaundice,   or icterus, is the yellowing of skin and whites of the eyes following the accumulation of bile products in the blood. May be due to **hepatitis** or **liver disease;** it may arise due to blockage of the bile duct with gallstones (*see* **gall-bladder disease**) or cancer of the bile-duct or neighbouring organs; it may be a transient complication of another disease (e.g., yellow fever or **pneumonia**); it may arise from chemical poisons or drug prescription; it may be a factor of some haemolytic blood diseases, pernicious anaemia, or faulty blood transfusions. It is a common and mostly harmless symptom in new-born infants.

---

jimson weed, Jamestown-weed, Thorn apple, Stramonium, *Datura stramonium* L. Fam: Solanaceae.

A coarse annual herb reaching 1 metre in height and as much in breadth with large angular leaves with deeply incurving toothed margins and pronounced reticular veins; white trumpet-shaped flowers up to 10cm long appear above a long green calyx in the leaf axils, giving way to a spiny capsule in shape similar to a horse chestnut which opens to reveal numerous dark seeds; the plant has a disagreeable odour.

Habitat: waste places, wood edges, roadsides throughout the world.

Constituents: tropane alkaloids (including hyoscine, hyoscamine and traces of atropine).

Actions: anticholinergic (i.e., bronchial and visceral antispasmodic, metabolic depressant, antibradycardic); variously sedating and stimulating the central nervous system.

Applications: to asthmatic conditions (most effectively when smoked but may be taken internally as well); to irritable, painful and intractable coughing; to the salivation and spasm of Parkinsonism.

Dosage: maximum permitted is 50mg of dried herb three times per day.

Caution: this remedy may be sold only to practitioners in the UK under the terms of the 1968 Medicines Act; taken in excess it produces cerebral depression, tachycardia, depressed respiration and coma. It must never be used in pregnancy, prostatic disease, tachycardia, glaucoma or with depressant drugs.

---

joe-pye weed, *see* **gravel root.**

Juglans cinerea, butternut.

---

juices, or succi, are preparations obtained by **expression** of fresh plant material.

---

juniper, *Juniperus communis* L. Fam: Coniferae.

The berries of a bush or tree of varying height, either prostrate or erect (up to 10 metres); needle-like leaves occur in whorls of three; the male plant bears a cone 1cm long, the female one of only a quarter that size; the fruit appears on the female plant, initially green, turning purplish-black in the second and third year on the plant.

Habitat: throughout the northern hemisphere from warm to polar regions, preferring heaths, moorlands and chalk downs.

Constituents: volatile oil (including pinene and camphine), resin, bitter principle (juniperin), antitumour agent (podophyllotoxin), flavonoids, tannins.

Actions: urinary antiseptic, diuretic, increasing elimination of acid metabolites, carminative and digestive tonic, stimulating uterine contractions.

Applications: to urethral, bladder and ureteral infections ('cystitis'); gouty and other arthritic conditions associated with accumulation of acid wastes; gastric conditions associated with reduced gastric secretions; colic and flatulent digestive problems.

Dosage: 1-2 grams of dried fruit equivalent three times per day.

Caution: not to be used where kidney disease is suspected and never during pregnancy.

Juniperus communis, juniper.

K

---

kava-kava, Ava, *Piper methysticum* Forster. Fam: Piperaceae.

The dried and peeled rhizome and roots of a shrub obtained commercially in chopped light yellow-brown pieces, longitudinally wrinkled with white circular root scars, breaking easily to reveal a pale interior; the odour is slight and the taste sweet, then strong followed by a slight numbness.

Habitat: South Sea islands.

Constituents: resin (including lactones kawahin, yangonin, methysticin), mucilage.

Actions: diuretic and urinary antiseptic; circulatory stimulant;

antispasmodic and analgesic (locally rubefacient and anaesthetic); mental stimulant in small doses, otherwise depressant.

Applications: to urinary, prostatic and vaginal infections; rheumatic conditions associated with urinary troubles, oliguria or water retention; locally for joint and muscle pains, used traditionally as a tonic in debility, especially when affecting sexual performance.

Dosage: 1-4 grams of dried rhizome and root equivalent three times per day.

---

kelp,   Bladderwrack, Black-tang, Rockweed, *Fucus vesiculosus* L. Fam: Fucaceae.

A familiar seaweed in the form of long ribbons or thalli, around 100cm long and 5cm across, leathery, shiny, olive-green to yellow-brown; down the centre of each thallus is a midrib on either side of which are the air-filled bladders which keep the seaweed (actually alga) floating up from its rocky anchorages. There are other so-called 'kelps' but this species is the only one described below.

Habitat: the coast of the Atlantic ocean and the Baltic, Irish and North seas; often washed up on beaches after storms.

Constituents: mucilage, pigments, fucosterin, fucoxanthin, zeaxanthin, iodine and many other minerals in large quantity.

Actions: gentle metabolic stimulant; nutritive; thyroid restorative; alterative.

Applications: to low metabolic rate, low thyroid activity, and other symptoms of a sluggish constitution; chronic joint and other inflammations in such conditions; thyroid disease of any description (as an **adaptogen**).

Dosage: 5-10 grams of the dried thallus equivalent three times per day.

---

kidney diseases,   conditions marked by any of a variety of symptoms, notably pain in the loins, blood, pus or protein in the urine, very scanty or very profuse flow. Causes include glomerulonephritis (or Bright's disease), tuberculosis, abscess, tumour, and **pyelonephritis** or pyelitis. All are potentially serious and complex and are not to be lightly treated, and as many herbs are likely to irritate a diseased kidney, this applies as much to the herbalist, unless well qualified to do so.

---

kola,   Cola, Guru nut, *Cola vera* Schum., *C. nitida* A. Chev., and *C. acuminata* Schott & Endl. Fam: Sterculiaceae.

The seeds of large trees (up to 12 metres), dark red-brown in colour, about 2-3cm across, plano-convex or irregular in shape, smooth and hard externally, with a pale-brown inner surface; the taste is slightly bitter and astringent.

Habitat: Sierra Leone, North Ashanti and around the Niger delta. Cultivated in the West Indies, Brazil and Java.

Constituents: alkaloids (including caffeine, theobromine), kola red, condensed tannins, volatile oil.

Actions: central nervous stimulant and tonic; astringent; diuretic.

Applications: to depressive conditions and nervous debility and exhaustion where a certain amount of stimulation is acceptable; diarrhoea and bowel looseness associated with debility, weakness or convalescence.

Dosage: 0.5-3 grams of dried powdered seeds equivalent three times per day.

Krameria triandra,   rhatany root.

L

---

labour,   it is an offence in the U.K. to attend a woman in childbirth without medical supervision unless a certified midwife or registered nurse; nevertheless, once labour contractions have commenced, it is possible that the woman herself would wish to take a herbal remedy to improve the efficiency of the birth process. Safe alternatives include raspberry leaves, beth root and squaw vine. The same remedies may be used after the birth to hasten elimination of the placenta and to stimulate healthy invôlution.

Lactuca virosa,   lettuce, wild.

---

ladies' mantle,   Lion's foot, *Alchemilla vulgaris* L. Fam: Rosaceae.

A low perennial herb with tufts of large orb or kidney-shaped leaves sharply divided into seven to nine broad, regularly toothed lobes, on long stalks; the low flowering stems bear loose panicles of small green flowers.

Habitat: in pastureland over northern Europe and Asia and over most of Britain and in eastern North America.

Constituents: tannins.

Actions: astringent, both locally, and apparently, systemically; regulatory on the menstrual cycle; digestive tonic; alterative.

Applications: to enteritis and resultant diarrhoea; to excessive menstrual bleeding; to excessive bleeding from any cause; locally for discharges and discharging wounds, especially as a douche.

Dosage: 1-4 grams of dried herb equivalent three times per day.

---

lady's slipper, American valerian, Nerve root, *Cypripedium pubescens* Willd. Also *C. parviflorum* Salisb. Fam: Orchidaceae.

The rhizome of an orchid with broad-veined leaves up to 15cm long; the flower has a large sac-like yellow 'slipper' with twisted pale-yellow-to-brown petals and sepals both striped with purple; the rhizome is externally rusty to brown, internally yellowish to white with a dense mat of roots underneath; the smell is faintly reminiscent of valerian, the taste bitter and acrid.

Habitat: in woods and thickets of North America; rare, but cultivated elsewhere.

Constituents: volatile oil, glycosides, resins and tannins.

Actions: sedative and antispasmodic; tonic to the nervous system.

Applications: to anxiety, neurosis, insomnia, restlessness, etc., particularly when associated with long-term debilitated conditions.

Dosage: 1-4 grams of dried root equivalent three times per day.

Lamium album, white deadnettle.

---

laryngitis, an inflammation and/or infection of the 'voice box' with hoarseness as the predominant symptom. Most often associated with upper respiratory conditions (*see* **catarrh** *and* **throat problems**), but may also coincide with lower respiratory disease, excessive use of the voice, alcohol and cigarette consumption and poor diet. Such background factors must therefore be assessed in treatment, and any ill health corrected. Specific treatment will be as for catarrh, throat problems and bronchial conditions, with particular emphasis on steam inhalations. Any case of laryngitis that persists for more than a few weeks should be referred for specialist diagnosis to exclude the possibility of growths forming.

Lavandula officinalis, lavender.

---

lavender, *Lavandula officinalis* Chaix., *L. vera* D.C., *L. spica* L. Fam: Labiatae.

The flowers of a perennial herb with crooked, branched woody stems, covered with flaky bark, giving off numerous straight, slender, four-sided stems with opposite, narrow, pale leaves with turned down margins; the flowers are produced in whorls on the end of long spikes, purple-blue in colour; the scent is characteristic.

Habitat: native to southern Europe but grown widely, notably in southern France; traditionally the best scented were those grown in southern Britain.

Constituents: volatile oil (including linalyl acetate, linalool, geraniol, cineole, limonene).

Actions: relaxant and antispasmodic; circulatory stimulant; nervous tonic.

Applications: to nervous irritation, exhaustion and depression; digestive colic and flatulent dyspepsia; the oil used locally for headaches and arthritic pain.

Dosage: 0.5-2 grams of dried flowers equivalent three times per day.

---

laxatives, plants that actively promote bowel movements; most belong to the group **anthraquinone laxatives,** but many herbs have some effect in helping to move gut contents, including ash, blue flag, buckbean, burdock, butternut, celandine, dandelion, figwort, golden seal, heartsease and wild indigo; others are notably gentle and supportive and may be most freely used for all manner of bowel complaints (*see* **aperients**). In fact, the latter apart it is most important that the nature of the bowel sluggishness is understood before laxatives are prescribed (*see* **constipation**). The use of laxative remedies has been a central part of **eliminative** programmes, particularly in association with **cholagogues,** as it has long been appreciated that the bowel is one of the major sources of toxins, and that total transit time of gut contents is generally much longer in modern times than it used to be: bowel cleansing is particularly likely to be considered in catarrhal conditions and high blood pressure, as well as other conditions for which eliminative remedies are applied.

---

lemon balm, Balm, Honeyplant, *Melissa officinalis* L. Fam: Labiatae.

A mint-like plant well-known for its unmistakable scent; the leaves are bright green, the stems square, branching little at first but much more at the ends where the tiny white flowers grow out of the leaf axils. The roots of the plants do not 'creep' like the mints.

Habitat: native to southern, eastern and central Europe, widely grown around the world.

Constituents: volatile oil (including monoterpenes: citral, citronellal, geraniol, etc.); tannins; bitter principle.

Action: relaxant, equally effective in calming central nervous and digestive tensions.

Applications: to anxiety states, and the effect of excessive tensions; very effective for children's troubles; a pleasant and effective drink to be taken after a busy day and last thing at night; to relieve a range of dyspeptic conditions.

Dosage: 1-4 grams dried herb equivalent three times or more a day.

Leonurus cardiaca, motherwort.

Leptandra virginica, black root.

---

lettuce, wild, *Lactuca virosa* L. Fam: Compositae.

A biennial plant, growing up to 2 metres but usually much smaller, with an erect stem covered at the base with a few prickles and bearing above small bilobular leaves clasping the stem; there are numerous small, yellow composite flowers; the large radical leaves have bristles on the underside midrib; the whole plant yields a milky juice when freshly cut and tastes very bitter.

Habitat: southern and western Europe and northern Asia.

Constituents: latex ('lactucarium') containing bitters, lactucin, lactucone, lactupicrin, an alkaloid (possibly hyoscyamine), triterpenes (including lactucerol).

Actions: sedative; soothing, digestive tonic.

Applications: irritable and excitable conditions, especially where associated with poor digestive function; anxiety, manic states, neuroses as a mild sedative; as an aid in insomnia; to muscular or articular pains.

Dosage: 0.5-3 grams of dried leaves equivalent three times per day.

Caution: overdosage with this remedy will produce stupor, depressed respiration, coma and even death: it is to be used with respect.

Levisticum officinale, lovage.

---

licorice, *Glycyrrhiza glabra* L., *Liquiritia officinalis* L. Fam: Leguminosae.
The roots and stolons of a tall erect perennial with light, gracefully-spreading pinnate foliage with dark-green lanceolate leaflets that hang down at night; from the leaf axils grow long-stemmed spikes of numerous bluish-purple to white papilionaceaous flowers, followed by small leguminous smooth-skinned seed pods; the roots are brown, long and cylindrical, with fibrous longitudinally-striated cork and fibrous white to yellow interior; the taste is sweet and characteristic.

Habitat: a native of south-east Europe and south-west Asia to Iran, growing in open fields not far from running water; commercially cultivated until recently in northern England.

Constituents: glycoside (glycyrrhizin: calcium and potassium salts of glycyrrhizic acid), triterpenoid saponins, flavonoids (including liquiritigetol), bitter (glycyrmarin), volatile oil, oestrogenous substances (including beta-sitosterol), asparagin, coumarins, tannins.

Actions: having an ACTH-like action on the adrenal cortex, increasing the production of gluco- and mineralocorticoids; similar anti-inflammatory effects to hydrocortisone but inhibiting its antigranulomatous action and its effects in increasing liver glycogen storage; producing a highly viscous mucus over the stomach wall and reducing gastric acid secretion; an antipyretic effect comparable to sodium salicylate; increased excretion of bilirubin in the bile; visceral antispasmodic; relaxing **expectorant;** non-sucrose sweetener.

Applications: to gastric ulceration and inflammations; to adrenocortical insufficiency and as an instrument in the recovery from excessive steroid administration and the resulting adrenocortical depression; to respiratory infections and dry or asthmatic coughs; as a systemic anti-inflammatory; as a method for disguising the taste of medicines (but *see* **bitters**).

Dosage: 1-4 grams of the dried root equivalent three times per day before meals in neutral or alkaline solution.

Caution: although it is not definitely proven, there is the possibility that using licorice as a medicinal agent will tend to increase fluid retention and blood-pressure through an aldosteronic effect: its use in cases of hypertension should thus be discouraged and, in any case, close monitoring of blood pressure is strongly advised. For similar reasons there is a threat to blood potassium levels and its use with digitalis drugs should be discouraged.

---

life root, Golden groundsel, Squaw weed, Golden senecio, *Senecio aureus* L. Fam: Compositae.

A perennial herb up to 60cm high with slender, unbranched cottony stems, with lower leaves up to 15cm long and kidney-shaped, the upper leaves pinnatifid and much smaller; the yellow composite flowers are up to 2.5cm across; the taste is bitter.

Habitat: in wet ground throughout eastern North America.

Constituents: alkaloids (including senecifoline, senescine); possible saponin; resin.

Actions: uterine relaxant and tonic; stimulant to the gravid uterus; appearing to soothe and regulate in both nervous and vascular irritability.

Applications: to menopausal symptoms of nervous and emotional upset, and hot flushes, to some cases of dysmenorrhoea; to diminished menstruation.

Dosage: 1-4 grams of dried fresh herb equivalent three times per day.

Caution: not to be used in pregnancy.

---

lignum vitae, Guaiac, Guaiacum, *Guaiacum officinale* L., and *G. sanctum* L. fam: Zygophyllaceae.

The heartwood of an attractive evergreen tree reaching a height of 20 metres, with blue flowers; obtained commercially as greenish-brown pieces of very heavy wood (that sink in water), with slightly acrid taste and aromatic odour when warmed.

Habitat: West Indies, Florida and northern coasts of South America.

Constituents: resin acids, saponins (including guaiacosaponin), vanillin, polyterpenoid (guaiaguttin).

Actions: peripheral circulatory stimulant acting to reduce the need for the inflammatory response.

Applications: to chronic rheumatoid conditions and other inflammatory degenerative disease.

Dosage: 0.5-2 grams dried wood equivalent (best extracted in strong alcoholic tincture) three times per day.

Caution: to be avoided in hypersensitivity, allergic or acute inflammatory conditions.

Ligusticum levisticum, lovage.

---

lily-of-the-valley, May lily, May bells, *Convallaria majalis* L. Fam: Liliaceae.

The leaves of this small herb, arising from a creeping rootstock, around 10-15cm long with sheathed stalks; the leafless flowerstems support a one-sided spike of drooping, bell-shaped, white, sweet-scented flowers.

Habitat: in woodlands through Europe and Asia from the Mediterranean to the Arctic circle; cultivated and naturalized all over the world.

Constituents: cardioactive glycosides (including convallatoxin, convalloside, convallotoxol, convallotoxoloside, convallarin, convallamarin); saponins; flavonoids; asparagin.

Action: a digitalis-like stimulus to heart contraction, increasing myocardial efficiency and stroke volume without putting extra demands on coronary supply, and reducing excessive irritability of the myocardium; evidence suggests that the whole plant is more gradual in its effect than isolated digitalis glycosides, that it produces comparable effects with lesser dose, and that it is less neurotoxic, all the result of interaction between cardioactive glycosidal components; also diuretic.

Applications: to heart failure and cardiac arrhythmias.

Dosage: maximum permitted under the Act is 150mg of dried leaf equivalent three times a day.

Caution: the Medicines Act 1968 specifically confines the use of lily-of-the-valley to practitioners operating under the terms of that Act.

---

limeflowers, Lindenflowers, *Tilia europea* L., Fam: Tiliaceae.

An imposing tree recognized by the large, broadly ovate leaves and the graceful arching of its branches. The flowers are in cymes in groups of four to ten, pendulous, yellow-white, on long stalks arising from the centre of the large pale-green bracts. The flower with bract is used in medicine.

Habitat: as a specimen tree or in avenues in parks or gardens, and wild in woods and thickets in sunny positions throughout the temperate world.

Constituents: volatile oil, saponins, flavonoids, condensed tannins, mucilage.

Actions: **peripheral vasodilator,** relaxant, diaphoretic and diuretic; a suggested healing effect on blood vessel walls.

Applications: to cardiovascular conditions with a pronounced tension or anxiety factor, helping particularly with hypertension and atherosclerosis problems; as a gentle but effective relaxant especially for children and for those suffering from nervous irritability; as an important remedy for use in fever management.

Dosage: 1-4 grams of dried flowers equivalent three or more times a day.

---

linctus, a syrupy or mucilaginous liquid designed to be swallowed undiluted so as to provide a protective covering over the throat and oesophagus; *see* **demulcent.**

---

liniments, liquid or semi-liquid preparations for the skin, generally in an oily base; they are either **rubefacient,** or locally anaesthetic, in most cases, although soothing preparations are also possible; they may be either simply applied or massaged in.

---

linseed, Flaxseed, *Linum usitatissimum* L. Fam: Linaceae.

The seeds of a tall erect annual branched at the top with alternate erect narrow and sharp leaves 1-5cm long; rich blue flowers occur in a terminal cluster; the small seed is brown to yellow, oval, pointed at one end, about 4.5mm long and 2.5mm across with a mucilaginous and oily taste.

Habitat: a cultivated plant and weed of cultivation locally in England and throughout the world.

Constituents: 30-40 per cent fixed oil, mucilage, wax, glycoside (linimarin).

Actions: gentle bulk laxative; relaxing expectorant; locally drawing, soothing and healing.

Applications: to chronic or acute, atonic or spastic constipation; to soothe rasping, dry and irritable coughs; locally to draw boils and furunculoses and to ease chest pains of a bronchitic or pulmonary origin.

Dosage: 3-6 grams of the crushed seed equivalent three times per day.

Linum usitatissimum, linseed.

Liquiritia officinalis, licorice.

---

liver disease (chronic), any long-term disorder of liver function or damage to liver tissue, including the after effects of acute **hepatitis** and possible conditions associated with **gall-bladder disease;** it includes cirrhosis, primary biliary cirrhosis, chronic active hepatitis, as well as a wide range of poorly characterized conditions. Cancer of the liver or gall-bladder often involves special problems and is not to be included in the comments below. In any identified chronic liver disease, or even when there is reasonable suspicion of it because of previous disease or through exposure to toxic contamination, drug taking or pollutants, the herbalist adopts a long-term regime of herbs and diet. Remedies may be chosen from **hepatic, cholagogue** and **bitter** herbs, depending on circumstances, but always emphasizing the most gentle, such as dandelion and chicory root, artichoke and milk thistle seed. Because of the close connection between liver and bowel functions, it may also be advisable to provide **aperients** or **laxatives,** especially such as curled dock or rhubarb root (relying more on bitters and cholagogues if the bowels are already too loose). Dietary advice concentrates on providing high levels of fruit and raw vegetables, with good quality vegetable protein sources such as soya and other pulses, and potatoes. Of the fruit and vegetables, lemon and carrot are each in their own way specifically effective for the liver, and they may be taken juiced. All sources of fat, saturated or polyunsaturated, should be heavily restricted (this includes nuts and seeds). Alcohol, caffeine, smoking and unnecessary drug intake should be banned altogether. Occasional fasts under supervision can be a useful adjunct.

Apart from obvious liver disorders, many practitioners suspect reduced liver function in many diseases of immunological disturbance especially the **auto-immune diseases,** migraine, and the hypersensitivity or **allergy** diseases. They see the liver as particularly vulnerable to harm in the modern contaminated and polluted environment: it is thus often treated as described above in a wide range of apparently unrelated conditions.

Lobaria pulmonaria,   lungwort.

---

lobelia, Indian tobacco, Pukeweed, *Lobelia inflata* L. Fam: Lobeliaceae.

An erect annual with an angular hairy stem reaching 50cm in height giving off pale-green ovate or lanceolate leaves up to 7cm long with irregularly toothed margins, the teeth bearing tiny white warts; racemes of two-lipped, pale-blue flowers arise from slender stems from the upper leaf axils; they give way to inflated fruit capsules each containing numerous brown reticulated seeds; the taste is acrid.

Habitat: fields and cultivated ground in the eastern North America.

Constituents: alkaloids (lobeline, isolobinine, lobelanidine, lobinaline); bitter glycoside (lobelacrin); pungent volatile oil (lobelianin); resin; gum.

Actions: a relaxing and diffusive influence in inflamed, febrile, hypersensitive and irritable conditions of the body; stimulating expectorant (emetic in large doses), yet with antispasmodic action.

Applications: to asthmatic conditions and chronic bronchitis; as a constituent of prescriptions designed to manage or contain acute inflammatory, allergic, or hypersensitivity syndromes, and in fever management; locally to muscle spasms and rheumatic joints; an extremely highly regarded remedy by the **physiomedicalists;** has been used to help reduce nicotine addiction.

Dosage: maximum permitted dose is 200mg of dried herb equivalent three times per day; recommended dose is 20-50mg.

Caution: although toxicity of this remedy is not established, the presence of the nicotine-like alkaloid lobeline has led to its control under the terms of the 1968 Medicines Act in the U.K. It is not permitted to be sold to the general public.

Lobelia inflata, lobelia.

---

lotion, a non-oily liquid for application to the skin, or as washes for body apertures; they may be simple infusions or decoctions, or may be distilled spirits or even **tinctures;** gum tragacanth may be used as a thickening agent where required; lotions may be primarily **astringent, demulcent** or **antiseptic;** *see also* **ulcer (mouth), throat problems, gum disease, ear problems, eye problems, vaginal problems.**

---

lovage, *Levisticum officinale* Koch., *Ligusticum levisticum* L. Fam: Umbelliferae.

The roots of a large umbelliferous perennial with thick, fluted, hollow stem ascending up to 1.5 metres with large leaves divided into wedge-shaped segments; the umbels of yellow flowers produce elliptical curved fruits with three prominent winged ribs; the root is thick and fleshy, grey-brown on the outside, almost white internally; the whole plant has a strong odour like celery and angelica, with a warm and aromatic taste.

Habitat: indigenous to mountainous districts of southern Europe; naturalized elsewhere.

Constituents: volatile oil (including terpineols: angelic acid, carvacrol, phthalidene); coumarins; furanocoumarins (including psoralen); benzoic acid; sitosterols; resins; bitter principle; malic acid.

Actions: warming digestive tonic and carminative; antispasmodic; diaphoretic; soothing expectorant and anticatarrhal.

Applications: to flatulent and colicky digestive disturbances and poor appetite; bronchial infections and irritations; to painful and diminished menstruation; locally, as a mouthwash and gargle for mouth and throat problems.

Dosage: 0.5-2 grams of dried root equivalent three times per day.

---

lozenges, a dried, compressed and moulded, or cut, blend of medicinal agents in gum acacia, sugar and a liquid like rosewater; designed to be held in the mouth and dissolved slowly so mostly applied to **throat problems;** unsuitable for obnoxious tasting herbs.

---

lucerne, Alfalfa, Purple Medick, *Medicago sativa* L. Fam: Papilionaceae.

A perennial erect herb with leaves divided into three long-toothed leaflets, with stipules adhering to the leafstalks; close racemes of violet or blue flowers give way to a spirally twisted pod.

Habitat: cultivated and as an escape all over the world.

Constituents: alkaloids (asparagine, trigonelline); phytoestrogens (formometin, coumestrol); minerals and vitamins.

Actions: nutritive.

Applications: to convalescence and debility; to reduce haemorrhage and as a tonic after blood loss and during anaemia.

Dosage: 3-10 grams of dried herb equivalent three times per day.

---

lungwort, Lungmoss, Oak lungs, Tree lungwort, *Lobaria pulmonaria* (L) Hoffm., *Sticta pulmonaria* (L) Hook. Fam: Stictaceae.

A lichen with wide leafy thallus, divided and apparently cut off at the ends, with wavy margins, green-brown, the surface in dips and ridges, the underside with variegated colouring reflecting the contours; the taste is mucilaginous and bitter.

Habitat: on old trees and mossy rocks throughout Britain and Europe.

Constituents: mucilaginous principles (including arabitol), sterols, unsaturated fatty acids.

Applications: to irritable respiratory conditions, such as asthma and children's coughs; locally healing and soothing.

Dosage: 1-3 grams of dried lichen equivalent three times per day.

Note: lungwort herb, consisting of the dried leaf of *Pulmonaria officinalis* L., of the borage family with characteristically variegated leaves, and two to three coloured flowers, found in chalky soils in shady areas through Britain, Europe and west Asia, has many of the same uses, although it is more astringent in character and has an extra anticatarrhal action.

---

lymphatic, a remedy that appears to help the tissue-cleansing action of the lymphatic system; they are most likely to be applied traditionally to infective or inflammatory conditions resulting in enlarged lymph nodes ('glands'), but there is a widespread agreement that they have application to a broader range of toxic problems, as **eliminative** remedies, where there are signs that the lymphatic system is involved. Lymphatic remedies include the following: marigold, cleavers, wild indigo, poke root, queen's delight and fenugreek.

M

Ma-huang, *see* **ephedra.**

malaria, common in tropical areas, a feverish condition transmitted by mosquitoes, seen in non-tropical areas as recurrent relapses in sufferers returned from endemic areas; herbs that have been used with success include chinchona bark, chiretta and barberry bark.

marigold, Pot marigold, Mary bud, *Calendula officinalis* L. Fam: Compositae.

The bright orange flowerheads of an annual plant with angular branched stems and prominent pale-green spatulate or oblanceolate sessile leaves with widely spaced teeth, the whole plant between 30 and 60cm in height; the flowers are borne on an elegant crown-shaped receptacle, and as the petals drop off, a circular corona of seeds remains; this wild plant should be distinguished from the many cultivated marigolds, many of which come from different genera entirely.

Habitat: a native of Egypt and the Mediterranean area, now escaped from cultivation throughout temperate regions of the world, being easily naturalized; it prefers previously cultivated positions.

Constituents: carotenoids (pro-vitamin A), resin, essential oil, sterols, flavonoids, bitter principle.

Actions: a non-tannin astringent, anti-inflammatory, antispasmodic, local tissue healer.

Applications: to damaged or ulcerated gastric mucosa; aphthous ulcers, gum disease and pharyngeal infections as a mouthwash or gargle; locally for varicose and crural ulcers, haemorrhoids, anal fissures, and capillary haemorrhages; infective conditions marked by lymph node enlargement; as a constituent for eyebaths for conjunctival affections.

Dosage: 1-4 grams of dried flowerheads equivalent three times per day.

Marrubium vulgare,   horehound, white.

Marsdenia condurango,   condurango.

---

marshmallow,   Guimauve, Mallards, Schloss tea, *Althaea officinalis* L. Fam: Malvaceae.

The root and leaves of this erect perennial herb related to the hollyhocks; the flowering stems reach up to 120cm high, with stalked three- to five-lobed pale-green velvety leaves; the attractive pale-pink-to-white flowers with red united stamens grow on short stalks in the upper axils; the root is greyish-white externally, revealing when peeled a fibrous white structure with deep longitudinal furrows. Leaves and root have a pronounced mucilaginous quality on chewing and a mawkish-sweet taste.

Habitat: originally in salty marshes or wet or brackish uncultivated ground in southern Europe and northern Asia, now established through southern Britain and Europe, Australia and eastern North America.

Constituents: mucilage (35 per cent in the root, approximately 10 per cent in leaves); asparigin; tannins; phytosterol.

Actions: demulcent on exposed epithelial and mucous surfaces, notably the skin, mouth and digestive tract; acts by reflex (*see* **mucilages**) to loosen tight coughs and bronchial tension, and to calm urinary inflammation and spasm; diuretic.

Applications: to soothing external wounds and burns as a local application; soothing stomach and small intestinal inflammation (e.g., gastritis, peptic ulceration, enteritis), reducing the symptoms of hiatus hernia and oesophagitis; to loosen a tight dry cough; soothing curative influence on inflamed urinary passages (e.g., in cystitis or the symptoms of urinary stones).

Dosage: 2-6 grams of dried root or leaf equivalent three or four times per day.

---

maté,   Paraguay tea, Yerba maté, Jesuit's Brazil tea, *Ilex paraguariensis* St. Hil. Fam: Aquifoliaceae.

The leaves of a large shrub, glossy dark-green when fresh, about 6-12cm long, that are quickly dried over wood fires and chopped up and often ground to produce fragments of pale green-brown leathery leaf and powder; the taste is bitter and astringent.

Habitat: Brazil, Paraguay and Argentina, originally near streams.

Constituents: alkaloids (including caffeine), tannins, volatile oil.

Actions: central nervous stimulant but with some calming properties; antispasmodic; diuretic.

Applications: nervous headaches associated with fatigue; to help control excessive appetite; when taken during the day to help induce a restful sleep at night.

Dosage: 1-4 grams of dried leaf equivalent three times per day.

Caution: like all caffeine-containing drinks, maté tea should be used in moderation.

Matricaria recutita et spp,   chamomile, wild.

---

meadowsweet,   Queen of the Meadow, Bridewort, *Filipendula ulmaria* L., *Spiraea ulmaria* L. Fam: Rosaceae.

The flowers and leaves of a striking plant easily recognized by its scented blooms, large, dense cymes of small, creamy-white regular bisexual flowers; these arise on stiff, reddish stems between 60 and 150cm high so tending to stand proud of surrounding vegetation; the leaves are characteristic in appearance, arranged as pairs of serrate leaflets of 1-7cm with very small ones at irregular intervals between, the terminal leaflet usually being three-lobed. The flowers have a light and pleasant fragrance.

Habitat: in damp places throughout Britain, Europe and central Asia, and the eastern half of North America.

Constituents: salicylic glycosides (spiraein, salicin, gaulterin); tannin; mucilage; flavonoids; volatile oil.

Actions: soothing and healing to the gastric mucosa, also reducing gastric acidity; diuretic, diaphoretic, antiseptic in acid conditions, anti-inflammatory; astringent.

Applications: to damaged gastric mucosa associated with hyperacidity; to controlling rheumatic conditions; for ascites and oedematous conditions; as an effective agent in managing a fever; for urinary infections.

Dosage: 2-5 grams of dried flowers and leaves equivalent three times per day.

---

measles,   or morbilli, a highly contagious viral disease, usually occurring in epidemics, marked by heavy colds, blood-shot eyes sensitive to the light, a harsh dry cough, and a widespread blotchy rash beginning behind the ears; herbal treatment will concentrate on **fever management,** to contain the occasionally high fever, eyebaths (*see* **eye problems**), and **expectorants** (most appropriately of the relaxing variety: this will also help the **nausea** and **vomiting.** Possible complications should be watched out for, but will be reduced with proper herbal care.

Medicago sativa,   lucerne.

---

medical herbalism,   the term used to denote the professional practice of herbalism in the U.K., and one statutorily recognized in the Medicines Act of 1968. The practice of medical herbalism is monitored by the National Institute of Medical Herbalists (NIMH) which sets a minimum standard of training (four years) before allowing applicants to sit examinations for membership. There is not, so far, any formal State registration in the profession. Practitioners will apply a blend of modern and traditional diagnosis and treatment to the full range of health problems, always emphasizing the potential of plant remedies to help the body in its fight to overcome the disease, rather than attacking the symptom alone. *See also* **phytotherapy, physiomedicalism.**

Melissa officinalis,   lemon balm.

---

menopause,   the time during which the menstrual periods and hormonal cycles cease; normally with little trouble, but there may be quite severe emotional disturbances, nervous irritability or depression, weight gain and water retention and, most notably of all, hot flushes. The herbalist's priority is to encourage the body to proceed with the change as smoothly as possible, rather than relying on temporary, and often delaying, alleviation of hormone replacement therapy. Thus, helonias root is applicable as an ovarian tonic, and restoratives like agnus-castus, St John's wort, life root and oats may be appropriate. **Relaxants** will often suggest themselves, particularly chamomile and black haw. Any heavy menstrual bleeding for more than a few months, and any bleeding outside menstruation, should be checked before treatment.

---

menstrual disorders, disturbances of the interacting hormonal and ovarian functions that control the development of the ovum, ovulation and menstruation each month. May be due to hormonal, psychological, mechanical (inflammation, damage, tumours such as fibroids, cysts), circulatory or even nutritional factors. In any case it is important to assess which factors are most significant. The individual problems will be dealt with under separate headings (*see* **menstruation, heavy; menstruation, irregular; menstruation, painful; pre-menstrual tension**) but there are a few general points to make. Hormonal disturbances can arise in a large number of ways, and do not always primarily involve the sex hormones; they are the most common factors in menstrual disorders. Herbal practitioners generally use remedies with a normalizing action, like agnus-castus, helonias root, or with tonic effects like dong quai or damiana. Circulatory problems are also common, given the much lower levels of exercise and the more sedentary lifestyle of modern times, and exercises are often recommended, along with such remedies as blue cohosh, shepherd's purse, white deadnettle, and life root, where pelvic congestion seems a factor. Anaemia and poor circulation might be apparent and might suggest the use of parsley, dong quai, rosemary, and appropriate **circulatory stimulants.** Any infection, inflammation, cysts, fibroids or back trouble will obviously require special attention (*see* **pelvic inflammation, fibroids, cervical problems, vaginal problems**).

---

menstruation, heavy, excessive bleeding at period time, or menorrhagia. Of approximately four main types: (1) due to pelvic circulatory congestion, alleviated by exercises and such remedies as white deadnettle, shepherd's purse, and life root, and blue cohosh; (2) due to capillary fragility, anaemia and associated vascular deficiencies, alleviated by parsley, buckwheat, limeflowers, yarrow; (3) due to inflammatory conditions of the pelvic organs (*see* **pelvic inflammation**); and (4) due to poor hormonal control of the latter part of the previous cycle (*see* **premenstrual tension**). Symptomatic remedies to control excessive menstrual bleeding include beth root, ladies' mantle, black haw, periwinkle, shepherd's purse and cranesbill.

---

menstruation, irregular, a category that can cover a number of conditions, including loss of periods (amenorrhoea), bleeding outside the normal time (metrorrhagia), as well as simple irregularity. By far the most common disruptions to menstrual cycles are **pregnancy** and **menopause**; the first of these must be positively eliminated before treating the condition further, whilst the possibility of menopause may be borne in mind in any woman over 37 or 38 and assumed when over 42 years of age. The next most common cause of amenorrhoea is nervous or nutritional stress, and the after effects of the contraceptive pill, hormonal or other drug treatment. In such cases and in most others where the cause is not apparent, uterine stimulants such as mugwort, southernwood, blue cohosh, parsley, cotton root bark or rue may be used, or such tonics as helonias root, dong quai, motherwort or life root may be preferred. Similar measures may also be appropriate in cases of irregular periods. Bleeding outside periods, whether flooding or spotting, demands a close examination of the health of the reproductive structures, as the most common causes are inflammation or other lesion in uterus, fallopian tube, cervix or vagina. Reference should be made to the appropriate area for treatment.

---

menstruation, painful, or dysmenorrhoea, traditionally is divided into two main groups: spasmodic and congestive. Spasmodic dysmenorrhoea is that most seen in early periods of adolescence and up to the first pregnancy, and typically starts with the first day of bleeding; it tends to be sharp and colicky; it appears to be associated with a combination of factors including relative excess of progesterone, high cervical tone, autonomic nervous and prostaglandin imbalance (as probably exacerbated in emotional tension). Prime remedies include cramp bark, black haw, blue cohosh, pasque flower, chamomile, white deadnettle and squaw vine, though other **relaxants** will often be indicated as well. Congestive dysmenorrhoea tends to be associated with premenstrual build-up and is often worst before menstruation; it tends to be dull and heavy and linked with water retention and other congestive signs; it may coexist with chronic **pelvic inflammation.** It is likely to respond over a period of some months to one or more of the following: agnus-castus, helonias root, parsley, dong quai, blue cohosh, white deadnettle and motherwort. In many cases treating the problem as an extension of **premenstrual tension** will be helpful. There are cases of dysmenorrhoea that do not fit neatly into the two categories, but from a herbal viewpoint they may usually be treated by appropriate blends of the above remedies, with additional recourse to **antispasmodics** where necessary.

Mentha piperita, peppermint.

Mentha pulegium, pennyroyal.

---

migraine,   an intense headache associated in many cases with digestive and visual disturbances, and often localized to one side of the head; of complex and shifting causes, but the headache produced by spasm of the blood vessels; can occur more or less regularly, often linked with hormonal cycles in women, or triggered by tension or rest from tension; treatment is always a complex affair. It is wise in the first instance to establish whether any migraine is a 'hot' or 'cold' type: the former is accompanied by excessive vasodilation and is relieved by the application of cold packs; the latter is accompanied by excessive vasoconstriction and is relieved by the application of hot packs (the majority are of this type). 'Hot' migraines are more likely to be helped by prescription that emphasizes the **bitter** (they are most likely to involve digestive or liver dysfunction) and **relaxant** or **sedative remedies.** 'Cold' migraines are most likely to be relieved by **circulatory stimulants** and **peripheral vasodilators** (like feverfew). **Hormonal remedies** are likely to be useful in many cases; **eliminative remedies,** especially **laxatives** may find their place; the possibility of food allergies should be investigated most closely. Temporary relief may be had where appropriate with valerian, gelsemium, Jamaican dogwood or wild lettuce; among the other remedies with reputations for positively helping migraine are rosemary, kola, lavender, vervain and feverfew. Each remedy and any other strategy should be carefully considered for its wider implications before being used, and quick changes in treatment are likely: especial care is often necessary to calm a sensitive stomach with **demulcents** before other remedies are given.

---

milk thistle,   *Silybum marianum* (L.) Gaertner., *Carduus marianus* L. Fam: Compositae.

The seeds of a biennial thistle, 60-90cm high with smooth leaves covered with variegated white veins, the lower leaves deeply pinnatified with broad, prickly lobes; there are large, drooping, solitary flowerheads with very prickly bracts; the seeds are pale brown to grey, about 7mm long, flattened, with a prominent callus at one end.

Habitat: dry and rocky waste places in southern and western Europe, locally in North America.

Constituents: flavonolignans (including silybin), flavonoids (including silymarin), bitter principle.

Actions: regenerating liver cells and protecting them against the action of liver poisons; stimulating bile flow.

Applications: to chronic liver disease and to aid rehabilitation after acute hepatitis; gall-bladder disease; whenever alcohol, drug or dietary abuse, or exposure to chemical pollution threatens normal liver function.

Dosage: 1-4 grams of dried seeds equivalent three times per day.

---

miscarriage, threatened, there have been a number of remedies traditionally used to reduce the chance of spontaneous abortion in vulnerable pregnancies; their use in modern times must be hedged about with caution and be subject to expert medical treatment. The following remedies may at least be considered in the appropriate circumstances; they are at least safe to take in pregnancy: black haw, helonias root, cramp bark.

---

mistletoe, Birdlime, *Viscum album* L. Fam: Lorantheaceae.

The stem and leaves of a parasitic evergreen found on trees, with green, forked stems and narrow, leathery leaves; the flower is small, yellow and unisexual, sitting in the fork of the stem, solitarily in the case of the female, and in clusters of three to five in the case of the male flowers. The female flowers give way to white berries containing one seed.

Habitat: throughout Europe, Asia and North Africa (the North American mistletoe is a completely different species), most commonly on oak, chestnut, black poplar and fruit trees, rarely on conifers.

Constituents: viscotoxin, saponins, alkaloids, tannin.

Actions: vasodilator; slowing and steadying an excessive heart rate; thus hypotensive; relaxant; diuretic; reputed antitumour activities.

Applications: to high blood-pressure, especially associated with nervous tension and high pulse rate; symptoms of nervous tension and spasm.

Dosage: 2-4 grams of the dried leaves and stems equivalent three times per day.

Caution: the berries of mistletoe are not permitted to be prescribed by anyone other than a registered medical practitioner under the terms of the 1968 Medicines Act; the rest of the plant is also coming under scrutiny on the basis of assumed dangers: none of these has yet been borne up by clinical experiment.

Mitchella repens, squaw vine.

---

morning sickness, nausea and vomiting during pregnancy, especially in the second and third months and not necessarily only in the morning. The benefit obtained from eating a dry biscuit or something sweet points the finger firmly at a low blood sugar level (*see* **hypoglycaemia**) and this may be the best angle to pursue; any other predisposing factor should be taken into account ; chamomile and black horehound may be tried as simple remedies. If these do not work, or if the problem extends past the third month, then referral will be necessary. Excessive vomiting, hyperemesis gravidum, is serious and must not be left untreated.

---

motherwort,   Lion's Ear, *Leonurus cardiaca* L. Fam: Labiatae.

An erect perennial herb standing 60-120cm high with prominent coarsely-toothed five- to seven-lobed leaves; whorls of white-to-pink flowers arise in the upper leaf axils; the calyx and later the seed case are notable for the border of prickly teeth; the odour is unpleasant.

Habitat: in waste places and hedgerows through northern temperate regions; common in Britain.

Constituents: alkaloids (including leonurine, stachydrine), bitter glycosides, tannins, volatile oil.

Actions: gentle uterine stimulant; relaxant; reputed cardiotonic; carminative.

Applications: for painful periods, especially where associated with anxiety and nervous tension, and for reduced periods and disturbed menstrual cycles generally, especially where womb contraction is painful or insufficient; supports the pregnant uterus and helps prepare it for labour contractions; for nervous tension generally, notably for palpitations and tachycardia.

Dosage: 1-4 grams of dried herb equivalent three times per day.

---

mouse-ear,   Pilosella, *Hieracium pilosella* L. Fam: Compositae.

A perennial herb with spreading tufts of leaves and leafy, barren shoots; the small, stalked, oblong or lanceolate leaves are green and sparsely hairy above, and white and downy below; small heads of pale-yellow flowers are often externally tinged with red.

Habitat: dry ground throughout Europe, northern Asia, and eastern and mid-North America; it is very common throughout Britain.

Constituents: umbelliferone, tannins, flavonoids, essential oil.

Actions: stimulating expectorant and healing of the respiratory mucosa; astringent.

Applications: to congestive and inflamed lung diseases, including whooping cough, and those causing traces of blood in the sputum, to provide substantial healing; as an astringent treatment to control the excesses of diarrhoea.

Dosage: 1-4 grams of the dried herb equivalent three times per day.

---

mucilages, complex carbohydrate constituents of many plants detected by their slimy quality in watery solution; their effect on the body is purely local, as they do not survive digestion and absorption into the body fluids. They act simply as **demulcent** and soothing agents, often having an incidental healing effect as well.

---

mugwort, *Artemisia vulgaris* L. Fam: Compositae.

An erect herb up to a metre in height with tough, grooved stems and many deeply pinnatifid leaves with five to seven lobes, dark-green above but silvery and hairy beneath; small, green-to-yellow, egg-shaped flowerheads crown the plant in long terminal spikes; the taste is bitter.

Habitat: common in waysides and waste places throughout temperate regions of the world.

Constituents: bitter glycosides (like wormwood), volatile oil, flavonoids, tannins.

Actions: stimulating delayed and inadequate menstruation; bitter stimulant of digestion.

Applications: to absent menstruation (but *see* **abortifacient**) and irregular and poor menstrual flow; as a bitter and antiseptic influence on the upper digestive tract (*see* **wormwood**).

Dosage: 0.5-2 grams of dried herb equivalent three times per day.

Caution: like all members of its genus mugwort is not to be used if pregnancy is suspected.

---

mullein, Aaron's rod, Lady's foxglove, Cow's lungwort, *Verbascum thapsus* L. Fam: Scrophulariaceae.

The flowers and leaves of a very tall, herbaceous biennial herb consisting of a rosette of very large, elongated, woolly, pale leaves, from the centre of which in the second year arises a tall, thick, tough stem, producing a dense terminal spike of five-petalled yellow flowers reaching as much as 3.5 metres in height.

Habitat: on dry banks and waste places throughout the whole temperate northern hemisphere.

Constituents: saponins (especially in the flowers), relaxing expectorant (leaves), demulcent.

Applications: to irritating inflammations of the trachea and bronchial tubes, with dry cough and/or bronchial spasm; for painful and hard

coughing; the flowers steeped in olive oil make excellent eardrops.
Dosage: 2-8 grams of dried leaves equivalent, or 1-2 grams of flowers, three times per day.

---

mumps,   or infectious parotitis, is a viral disease of glandular structures in the body, most often affecting the salivary glands in children and adolescents, but possibly also the testicles (orchitis) in post-adolescent males and rarely the ovaries (oophoritis) in women; marked by mild fever and sore throat followed by swelling of parotid gland in front of ear on one side, then the other; in children it is a mild condition requiring only sensible care (*see* **fever management**), and mouth washes with tinctures of thyme and other **antiseptic** herbs (*see* **throat problems**); in post-adolescents especially **lymphatic** remedies such as clivers, marigold and poke root will be indicated, as will **anti-infectives,** to reduce the risk of gonadal involvement and even possible infertility.

---

myalgia,   sometimes known as 'muscular rheumatism', fibrositis or lumbago, and generally occurring in those past middle age, is inflammation of the connective tissues covering the muscles, and of the tendons. It has many similarities to, and may be treated in the same way as, **neuralgia,** but applied externally (*see* **rubefacients**); internal remedies most directly applicable to myalgia include buckbean, sweet chestnut, bryony, black cohosh, cinchona, wild yam and devil's claw, and there is often advantage in seeing the problem as a form of rheumatic condition (*see* **rheumatism**).

Myrica cerifera,   bayberry.

Myristica fragrans,   nutmeg.

---

myrrh,   *Commiphora molmol* Engl. Fam: Burseraceae.
   The resin of a bushy tree up to 3 metres in height with tough, knotted branches, and spine-tipped twigs sparsely covered with small, trifoliate, irregular leaves; the resin is obtained in irregular masses, yellow to red-brown, hard and brittle and tacky to the touch, translucent with white flaws and patches; the taste is acrid and bitter, the odour characteristic and aromatic.
   Habitat: in desert areas by the Red Sea shores of Saudi Arabia and in Somalia.

155

Constituents: resin (including commiphoric acids); volatile oil (including m-cresol, eugenol, formic acid, acetic acid, heerabolone); gum; bitter principle.

Actions: locally antiseptic, astringent and healing, provoking leucocytosis; expectorant and diaphoretic.

Applications: to infections and inflammations of the mouth, gums, throat and head area, including upper respiratory catarrhal conditions and the common cold; locally for wounds, ulcers, fungal infections.

Dosage: as a tincture only, the equivalent of 0.3-1 gram of resin three times per day.

N

---

nausea,   feeling queasy and sick and close to vomiting; due to reactions to foods, poisons and medicines, even herbal; or to **stomach problems;** also nervous tension, **travel sickness, migraine, morning sickness, liver disease, food poisoning** and abdominal infections. After treatment of appropriate cause is undertaken, symptomatic relief may be had with Iceland moss, Irish moss, cassia, cinnamon, horehound (black), nutmeg or chamomile.

Nepeta cataria,   catmint.

Nepeta hederacea,   ground ivy.

---

nervine,   *see* **nervous restoratives.**

---

nervous bowel,   a state of overactivity of the large intestine or colon. Often ascribed, wrongly, as an entirely psychological problem. In fact due to a tendency to transfer tensions onto the system co-ordinating bowel movements so that the latter 'picks up' any tensions the sufferer encounters. Symptoms include alternating diarrhoea and constipation, or either alone, frequent bowel urges, the passage of mucus (hence 'mucous colitis'), and abdominal discomforts. Best treated with a course of **relaxants,** notably chamomile, hops, wild yam, and the carminatives like fennel or dill, so as to allow the natural rhythm of the bowel to reassert itself free from extraneous interference. A natural pattern may thus be established eventually without treatment. *See also* **diarrhoea.**

---

nervous breakdown,   a crescendo of psychological and nervous tensions leading to a collapse in the sufferer's ability to carry on a normal routine; by its nature difficult to predict, or treat until after it has happened; then **nervous restoratives** may be applied as remedies, and a programme of **convalescence** instituted. As always any relevant background factor can be treated as appropriate. (*See also* **nervous problems.**)

---

nervous problems,   in herbal terms the nervous system is seen as an intrinsic part of the whole body's functions; while it is clearly the seat of a completely different level of experience, as far as herbal treatment is concerned, nervous disturbance is likely to have somatic implications, and it is more than possible that somatic disturbances are actually predisposing to nervous disorders. Thus neuroses, phobias, depression, and even psychoses like schizophrenia, may be partially corrected at root by the use of **nervous restoratives** and **relaxants,** and by attention to any outstanding dysfunction elsewhere in the body. In traditional medicine nervous problems would come within the remit of the shaman or witchdoctor, and from time to time psychoactive herbal remedies such as cannabis, yohimbe, cola, peyote, coca, opium poppy, ergot, jimson weed, tobacco and wild lettuce, have been used as part of a healing ritual combining elements of myth and other collective symbols in a spiritual, emotional and psychological catharsis. Such traditional forms of psychotherapy do not translate well to the modern environment, and the use of most psychoactive agents is limited by law. It must however be said that there is a potential for the careful development of treatment using such herbs as key agents by suitably qualified therapists.

---

nervous restoratives,   remedies that are used to restore the nervous system in debility, appearing to have something of a nourishing function; used by herbal practitioners instead of **stimulants** in fatigue, nervous exhaustion, mental depression, and even such nervous affections as **shingles, neuralgia** and multiple sclerosis, as well as other neurological disease, psychoses and any disease that involves the nervous tissues (*see* **nervous problems**). The action of the nervous restoratives is generally slow but steady, providing for a genuine improvement in tone of the nervous tissues over weeks or months. Notable examples are oats, damiana, St John's wort, vervain, (Asiatic) ginseng, gotu kola, rosemary, scullcap, lavender, lady's slipper, squaw vine and kola (with discretion). Some of these are also **relaxant,** others more stimulating, and these qualities will significantly affect their application. In any restorative regime for the nervous system it is always wise to consider the potential for **circulatory stimulants.**

---

nettle, Stinging nettle, (1) Common perennial nettle, *Urtica dioica* L., (2) annual nettle *U.urens* L. Fam: Urticaceae.

Well-known plants notable for their painful stings; there are two species used medicinally, the commoner perennial form with creeping invasive rootstock and coarse foliage with downy covering over the whole plant; the smaller annual species, rarely over 30cm high, has more delicate smooth shiny foliage and no large rootstock; in the latter case the small bisexual flowers are almost sessile, in the perennial form stalked.

Habitat: as a common weed of cultivation, the annual nettle more likely in the fields and gardens themselves, the perennial form in waste ground and long-neglected areas.

Constituents: acrid components (in the stinging hairs: including formic acid, histamine, volatile and resinous acids); silica; glucoquinone; tannins; large quotas of minerals and vitamins (like all voracious plants robbing the soil of minerals).

Actions: nutritive; haemostatic and astringent; circulatory stimulant; diuretic; galactogogue; hypoglycaemic.

Applications: to skin disease associated with poor peripheral circulation and/or anaemia; infantile and allergic eczema; melaena; uterine haemorrhage; gout and other cases of uricosaemia; as an aid in late-onset diabetes mellitus; to promote milk production in humans and animals.

Dosage: 2-4 grams of dried herb equivalent three times per day.

---

nettlerash, hives, or urticaria, is an allergic reaction manifested as itchy swellings on the skin, sometimes leading to blistering but most often of a very transient nature. Can be part of a wider allergic condition (*see* **allergy**), or a simple reaction to an item of diet or environment. Only rarely is it serious, but digestive function may be central and should be treated if the condition is persistent.

---

neuralgia, painful inflammation of nerve fibres, likely to arise anywhere but notably in the trigeminal nerve of the face (trigeminal neuralgia: 'tic douloureux'); marked by often severe pain that is usually exacerbated by cold and draughts. From the herbalist's point of view, the condition marks a debility, especially of the nervous system, and calls for treatment with **nervous restoratives** and **circulatory stimulants.** **Analgesic** remedies may be used selectively, and **relaxants** will often be useful. There is often advantage in using local applications such as lavender oil, wintergreen oil and poultices of linseed. *See also* **myalgia.**

---

neurosis, *see* **nervous problems.**

---

night sweats, *see* **perspiration, excessive.**

---

nutmeg, *Myristica fragrans* (Houtt). Fam: Myristicaceae.

The kernels from a tree reaching about 8 metres in height; the kernels are about 3cm long by 2cm broad; pale-brown with a network of grooves and lines; the transverse section shows the pale-brown endosperm penetrated by numerous infoldings of darker perisperm; the odour and taste are aromatic and characteristic.

Habitat: indigenous to the islands of South-East Asia; also grown in the West Indies.

Constituents: volatile oil (including pinene and eugenol), fixed oil ('nutmeg butter'), with small amounts of myristicin and safrol.

Actions: carminative; antispasmodic; prostaglandin-inhibiting anti-inflammatory; digestive tonic and gastric stimulant; cerebral stimulant.

Applications: to flatulent nervous dyspepsia; nausea and vomiting; intestinal spasm, colic and flatulence; inflammatory disease of the gut wall.

Dosage: 0.3-1 gram of dried kernel three times per day.

Caution: larger doses are dangerously stimulating to the central nervous system.

Nymphaea odorata, white pond lily (American).

O

oak bark, Tanner's bark, *Quercus robur* L. *et spp.* Fam: Fagaceae.
The bark of the familiar tree, obtained in cut pieces with silvery-grey cork externally marked with brown lenticels, internally brown or red-brown with longitudinal striations, with fibrous fracture; the taste is very astringent.
Habitat: indigenous to Britain, Europe and North America.
Constituents: condensed and hydrolysable tannins.
Actions: strongly astringent.
Applications: to acute diarrhoea, to control the loss from the bowel; locally as a mouthwash and gargle for discharging, bleeding or infected surfaces of the mouth and throat; as a local application for haemorrhoids; as a douche for cervical and vaginal discharges.
Dosage: 0.5-2 grams of dried bark equivalent three times per day.

---

oats, *Avena sativa* L. *et spp.* Fam: Gramineae.
The whole oat plant cropped when the seeds are ripe is the best form of this remedy (sometimes called oatstraw in this case); wild oats are as good as the commercially cultivated varieties; oatmeal is a good second best.
Constituents: saponins, alkaloids (including avenine and trigonelline), a sterol, flavonoids, silica, calcium and many other minerals, wheat protein (gluten).
Actions: a sure and effective restorative to the nervous system.
Applications: for all states of debility, particularly involving the nervous system, to take in conditions such as depression, 'neurasthenias', shingles and other herpes infections, and even the degenerative wasting conditions such as multiple sclerosis. In such cases the remedy exerts a gentle but solid restorative action, making substantial contributions to tissue health.
Dosage: 1-4 grams dried herb or oatmeal equivalent three times per day.
Caution: the presence of gluten may provide problems in those conditions that arise from gluten sensitivity (some cases of multiple sclerosis for example). This can be eliminated by making a decoction or tincture, allowing to settle and carefully decanting the clear liquid off the solid material.

Oregon grape, Mountain grape, Holly-leaved barberry, *Berberis* *aquifolium* L. Fam: Berberidaceae.

The rhizome and roots of a shrub up to 2 metres in height, with shiny compound leaves and with yellow-green flowers in loose terminal racemes giving way to purple berries; the rhizome is obtained in cylindrical pieces, externally yellow-brown, internally bright yellow and with prominent rays; the taste is bitter.

Habitat: the west coast of North America; cultivated elsewhere as an ornamental.

Constituents: alkaloids (including berberine, oyacanthine, herbamine).

Actions: cholagogue and mild laxative, generally used as an alterative; digestive stimulant and tonic.

Applications: to skin, joint and other inflammatory disease associated with hepatic, digestive and bowel defects.

Dosage: 0.5-2 grams of dried rhizome and root equivalent three times per day.

---

osteoarthritis,   a disease of the joints, generally brought about in those subject to excessive wear and tear, e.g., the weight-bearing joints of knee, hip, ankle and spine, or those of the hand in particular occupations; a wearing and erosion of the protective cartilage is combined with inflammatory attack to lead to progressive breakdown of the joint, with pain and disability. General measures should be to avoid excessive strain of the affected joint, though exercise as such is useful (walking and standing are bad: swimming and floor exercises are good). Herbal remedies are chosen for their apparent ability to cleanse the joints of unnecessary accumulations that in turn provoke inflammation; they include celery seed, lignum-vitae, juniper, wall germander and devil's claw; **circulatory stimulants** and **diuretics** are also likely to be well favoured; for dietary and other advice *see* **arthritis**.

---

otitis,   *see* **ear problems.**

P

palpitations, alarming but harmless awareness of the heart pounding, in reality a form of 'resonance' highlighting normally unconscious heartbeat. Brought on in states of nervous tension, debility, acute disease, dyspepsia, over-consumption of tea, coffee or alcohol, and sudden emotional shock. The first priority is to reassure the sufferer that the symptoms are not serious, and to prescribe peace and quiet; any underlying causes should be treated directly; herbal **relaxants** are of great use, and limeflowers are almost specific.

Panax ginseng, ginseng, Asiatic.

Panax quinquefolium, ginseng, American.

---

pansy, wild, *see* **heartsease.**

Parietaria diffusa et spp, Pellitory-of-the-wall.

---

parsley, *Petroselinum crispum* Mill., *Carum petroselinum* Benth & Hooker., *P. sativum* Hoffm. Fam: Umbelliferae.

The well-known kitchen-garden herb grown for its curly, pinnate segmented leaves for use as a garnish and flavouring. It is a biennial, so flowering and seeding in its second year. The seeds, root and leaves are all used.

Habitat: indigenous to countries around the eastern Mediterranean, now grown and naturalized throughout the world, naturalizing especially to maritime areas and limestone and rocky locations.

Constituents: volatile oil (including apiol — 'parsley camphor'); begapten; flavonoid (apiin); fatty oil; large quantities of vitamins C and A; and minerals, iron, calcium, phosphorus and manganese.

Actions: strong diuretic, carminative and digestive tonic, antispasmodic, stimulant of uterine muscle, nutritive.

Applications: to urinary infections and calculi; oedematous conditions;

depressed gastric and digestive performance; visceral and vascular spasms; for post-natal womb involution and the promotion of lactation; for arthritic conditions linked to defective kidney eliminations; to anaemic and debilitated conditions as a long-term dietary supplement (the leaves are best for this last effect).

Dosage: 1-4 grams of dried root or leaves (1-2 grams of seeds) equivalent three times per day.

Caution: the seeds and heavy consumption of the herb are to be avoided in pregnancy.

---

parsley piert, Parsley breakstone, *Aphanes arvensis* L. *Alchemilla arvensis* Scop. Fam: Rosaceae.

A small, much-branched green annual herb 2-7cm high, covered in soft hair; sharply divided leaves on short stalks with tiny green sessile flowers in their axils.

Habitat: stony ground, old walls and such areas through Britain, Europe and western Asia.

Constituents: not established with any certainty.

Actions: diuretic and soothing to the urinary mucosa.

Applications: to urinary calculi and associated problems

Dosage: 2-4 grams of dried herb equivalent three times per day.

---

parturifacient, a remedy that improves the efficiency and reduces the time, discomfort and complications of labour (*see* **labour**).

---

pasque flower, Pulsatilla, Wind flower, Meadow anemone, Prairie anemone, *Anemone pulsatilla* L. Fam: Ranunculaceae.

The long-stalked leaves of a perennial herb, covered at first with silky hairs and divided into long, thin segments; the flowerstalks are 12-20cm high and end in a prominent solitary purple flower made up of six silky sepals with the inner involucre projecting increasingly forward as the flower ripens.

Habitat: limestone pastures in central and northern Europe and locally in southern Britain.

Constituents: glycoside (ranunculin in the fresh plant converting to anemonin when dried), saponins, tannins, resin.

Actions: calming and sedative, with particular application to pain and inflammation in the reproductive system.

Applications: to painful menstruation associated particularly with reduced flow; to inflammation and infection of male or female reproductive organs and tissues; to nervous tension and anxiety, particularly of menopause or premenstrually.

Dosage: 0.2-0.3 grams of dried leaves equivalent three times per day.

Caution: the fresh plant must not be used, and even the dried plant should be used only with care (*see below*).

Passiflora incarnata, passionflower.

---

passionflower, Grenadille, Maypop, *Passiflora incarnata* L. Fam: Passifloraceae.

The aerial parts (collected after harvesting) of a herbaceous perennial climbing plant with three-lobed finely toothed leaves, and bare shoots producing the decorative purple-tinged yellow or pink flowers giving way to the orange berry known as passionfruit.

Habitat: south-east North America; cultivated in southern Europe and western South America.

Constituents: alkaloids (including harmine, harman, harmol, passiflorine); flavonoids (including saponarin, saponetin, vitexin); sterols.

Actions: relaxing antispasmodic with some sedative properties; peripheral vasodilator.

Applications: to restlessness and irritability and insomnia arising out of such causes; conditions of high nervous or visceral tension or spasm.

Dosage: 0.5-1 gram of dried plant equivalent three times per day.

---

pastille, a softer form of **lozenge,** made with a glycerine and gelatine base and mostly used for problems of the mouth, gums and tongue, as well as throat.

---

pectoral, *see* **expectorant.**

---

pellitory-of-the-wall, *Parietaria diffusa* Mert & Koch., *P. officinalis* L. Fam: Urticaceae.

A small branching perennial initially growing erect but becoming procumbent when 15-30cm long, with alternate stalked ovate, downy leaves; unisexual flowers occur in very small sessile clusters, the male very indistinguishable, the female tubular and four-lobed.

Habitat: on old walls and stony ground throughout Britain, Europe and northern Asia.

Constituents: bitter glycoside, tannins.

Actions: diuretic and soothing to the urinary mucosa.

Applications: painful micturition, associated with infection or calculi; oedema associated with reduced micturition.

Dosage: 1-4 grams of dried herb equivalent three times per day.

---

pelvic inflammation (chronic), low-grade infection or inflammation of the pelvic organs, most often used to refer to such a case in the female, and infections of the fallopian tubes (salpingitis) and/or ovaries (oophoritis). Such inflammation may follow acute salpingitis (either from gonorrhoea, or following childbirth or abortion) or may result from the presence of the coil, or almost any other intervention or infection in the area. The symptoms are variable, but mostly include low backache especially just before menstruation and often associated with congestive **dysmenorrhoea,** pain at ovulation time, profuse and possibly frequent periods, persistent unpleasant discharge, and pain on deep penetration during intercourse. Infertility may be a prominent problem and is a growing risk as the disease persists. Treatment of this condition is best left to a qualified practitioner; helonias root with echinacea taken over several months is almost specific, these remedies combined with such as blue cohosh, wild indigo and beth root as indicated.

---

pennyroyal, *Mentha pulegium* L. Fam: Labiatae.

A prostrate branched perennial mint with small, smooth leaves and small flowers in dense axillary whorls with characteristic odour.

Habitat: wet ground around the Mediterrancan and into Europe and western Asia; scattered in Britain.

Constituents: volatile oil (including pulegone).

Actions: carminative, diaphoretic, uterine stimulant.

Applications: calming flatulence, colic and other dyspeptic conditions; for insufficient painful menstruation.

Dosage: 1-3 grams of dried herb equivalent three times per day.

· **Caution:** pennyroyal should not be used in pregnancy of when any delayed menstruation might denote pregnancy: it is as likely to damage the foetus as procure the abortion.

---

peppermint, *Mentha piperita* L. Fam: Labiatae.

The leaves of a member of the mint family, actually a hybrid between watermint and spearmint; of a typically mint-like appearance with smooth leaves which are often purplish and purple labiate flowers; the odour is characteristic and is the best way of distinguishing it from its near relatives.

Habitat: as garden escapes locally around Europe and the British Isles.

Constituents: volatile oil (including menthol), bitter principle, tannins.

Actions: carminative and antispasmodic for the gut with notable action for the lower bowel; peripheral vasodilator and diaphoretic with a paradoxical cooling effect; cholagogue and bitter.

Applications: calming digestive upsets (e.g., dyspepsia, excessive tendency to vomiting, spastic or nervous bowel, flatulence, colic, diarrhoea); for vomiting of pregnancy; for managing fevers, especially in the 'hot' stages (i.e., when the patient feels hot, restless and agitated).

Dosage: 1-4 grams of dried herb equivalent three times per day.

---

percolation, a process of **extraction** whereby the solvent is allowed to trickle slowly down through a powdered mass under the influence of gravity, to be filtered off and collected at the bottom; generally considered to be an excellent way to gain most efficient extraction.

---

period problems, *see* **menstrual disorders.**

---

peripheral vasodilator, a term applied to remedies that dilate blood supply to the tissues, encouraging circulation without apparently stimulating it actively like the **circulatory stimulants,** classified in Galenic terms as 'hot in the first degree', they were seen then to normalize body temperature effectively, cooling it when it was too hot (*see* **fever management**), and warming it when cold (although **circulatory stimulants** would be more appropriate in practice); many of these remedies are also **diaphoretics** and thus find extra application in fevers; in clinical practice the peripheral vasodilators are used to improve the circulation in **arteriosclerosis, Raynaud's disease, Buerger's disease, chilblains,** and other conditions of poor circulation; for skin disease or in fact any inflammatory condition marked by evidence of poor circulation; to 'cold' **migraine;** to high blood-pressure. Examples of peripheral vasodilators are: yarrow, elderflowers, rosemary, hyssop, sage, feverfew, limeflowers, peppermint, prickly ash, hawthorn, boneset, chamomile, ephedra, garlic, ginger, sassafras, stone root, lignum-vitae, snake root, ammoniac, pleurisy root, ipecacuanha, gelsemium, quebracho, (Siberian) ginseng, black cohosh, buckwheat. Many of these are notable for other therapeutic effects: their peripheral vasodilatory action is in such cases generally taken as an important component of their total action on the body.

---

periwinkle, greater, *Vinca major* L. Fam: Apocynaceae.

A trailing plant with long slender stems occasionally re-rooting themselves and bearing pairs of opposite-pointed, glossy, dark-green leaves at intervals of around 2.5-4cm; a single pale blue flower grows up from each joint on a long stalk; the taste is bitter and astringent.

Habitat: woods and hedgerows, originally from southern Europe, but widely grown and naturalized throughout the world.

Constituents: alkaloids (including reserpine), tannins.

Actions: astringent; checking uterine haemorrhage.

Applications: to excessive menstrual bleeding and uterine discharge, both systemically and as a douche.

Dosage: 1-4 grams of dried herb equivalent three times per day.

---

perspiration, excessive, traditionally seen as a sign of debility, especially when occurring at night ('night sweats'); thus seen as an indication for restorative regimes, reduction in physical and mental strain and activity, and simple vegetable and fruit diets; **bitter** herbs may often be useful, depending on other indications, and sage, boneset, life root, and, when very severe, deadly nightshade for limited periods, can be used where appropriate. Excessive perspiration may also be a feature of **menopause**.

---

pessaries, solid preparations similar in basis to **suppositories,** but moulded so as to be applicable to vaginal insertion, thus providing a vehicle for the application of remedies for **vaginal problems**.

Petroselinum crispum, parsley.

Peumus boldo, boldo.

Phyllitis scolopendrium, Hart's-tongue fern.

---

physiomedicalism, a system of medical herbalism developed in the U.S.A. in the latter years of the 19th century, and imported to the U.K. before being legislated out of existence in the land of its birth. The basis of professional medical herbalism in the U.K. to this day. Evolving out of the populist movement initiated by Samuel Thomson in the early years of the century, which in turn was a blend of Indian herbal practice and the European settler tradition, physiomedicalism emphasized the role of the remedies in supporting the vital force, particularly in influencing circulation to various tissues, and in enhancing or controlling body functions. Physiomedicalism was a contemporary of ostcopathy and chiropractice and shares many of their orientations and aspirations; its value is still appreciated by practitioners and it is being re-worked as a substantial explanation of the unique qualities of herbal remedies in modern terms.

---

phytolacca americana et spp, poke root.

---

phytotherapy, a term used in continental Europe and increasingly in the U.K. to denote the use of plant remedies in medicine; favoured especially by those who wish to emphasize the modern potential of traditional remedies, and likely to feature more in scientific and legislative circles.

Picraena excelsa, quassia.

Picrasma excelsa, quassia.

---

piles, *see* **haemorrhoids.**

---

pilewort, Lesser celandine, *Ranunculus ficaria* L. Fam: Ranunculaceae.
The thick, dark-green, shiny, kidney-shaped leaves of a low perennial plant with annual creeping tuberous rootstock; the flower stems bear a single glossy yellow buttercup-like flower very early in the season.
Habitat: a common weed throughout Britain, Europe and western Asia.
Constituents: anemonin and protoanemonin.
Actions: locally astringent.

Applications: topically to haemorrhoids.
Dosage: Ointment BPC — 30 per cent fresh plant in benzoinated lard.
Caution: not recommended for internal consumption

---

pills, a coated or uncoated ball of herbs and other medicinal agents with binding agents or excipients, designed to hold together for dispensing but to dissolve easily in the stomach; now rarely made by the herbal practitioner, although still widely available on a commercial scale from major suppliers; a useful means of applying herbs especially those with an obnoxious taste, but inappropriate for those prescriptions relying on the **bitter** effect.

Pimpinella anisum, aniseed.

Piper methysticum, kava-kava.

---

pipsissewa, Prince's Pine, *Chimaphila umbellata* (L) Nutt. Fam: Pyrolaceae.
A small evergreen perennial with dark-green, leathery leaves with serrated margins growing in whorls from angular erect stems around 30cm high on a creeping or subterranean system of stems; flowers are single but borne in an umbellate inflorescence.
Habitat: dry woods through North America and northern Eurasia.
Constituents: arbutin, tannins, resin.
Actions: urinary antiseptic and diuretic; alterative.
Applications: to urinary infections and calculi; to arthritic and chronic inflammatory diseases linked to oedema; as a substitute for **uva-ursi.**
Dosage: 0.5-3 grams of dried leaves equivalent three times per day.

Piscidia erythraea, Jamaica dogwood.

Plantago lanceolata, ribwort.

Plantago major, plantain, greater.

Plantago ovata, psyllium.

Plantago psyllium, psyllium.

---

plantain, greater, Waybread, Rat's-tail plantain, Common plantain, *Plantago major* L. Fam: Plantaginaceae.

The leaves of a perennial herb, broad and ovate, up to 12cm long with around seven prominent ribs diverging from the broad footstalks; the flowerstalks are between 2 and 15cm long and bear a slender spike of tiny sessile flowers giving the characteristic 'rat-tail' effect.

Habitat: on roadsides and fields and wasteplaces all over the world.

Constituents: mucilage, glycosides (including aucubin), tannins, zinc and silica.

Actions: demulcent and astringent; relaxing expectorant; diuretic.

Applications: urinary tract infections and irritation; dry and nervous cough; gastric inflammation; locally for haemorrhoids.

Dosage: 1-4 grams of dried leaves equivalent three times per day.

---

plaster, the techniques of applying a fabric or other material binding to the skin was much used in former times as a vehicle for the application of **rubefacient, vesicant** or **healing** preparations; generally the herb or other material was impregnated with waxy or oily material into the fabric of the plaster and whole applied over the affected area.

---

pleurisy, infection and/or inflammation of the pleural membranes covering the lungs, generally as a secondary complication of other lung ailments or widespread illness; marked by sharp stabbing pain in one side of the chest aggravated by breathing, coughing or movement, possibly disappearing if there is effusion into the pleural cavity ('wet pleurisy'); there may be fever. Subject to expert advice about the need for antibiotics, or the presence of **tuberculosis,** herbal treatment will include soothing relaxing **expectorants** like pleurisy root, comfrey, mullein, thyme and licorice, warming remedies like garlic and ginger, **fever management** remedies as appropriate, and anti-infective remedies like echinacea and wild indigo. Pleurisy is a case where external application of herbs is very useful, and poultices of linseed, angelica leaf, and cabbage leaves are very likely to be useful. Occasionally in a particularly severe form of pleurisy, empyema, marked by pus in the pleural cavity with high fluctuating fever, can occur, and will require full medical attention.

---

pleurisy root, White root, Butterfly weed, Orange milkweed, Wind root, *Asclepias tuberosa* L. Fam: Asclepiadaceae.

The root of a handsome perennial plant growing to 50cm with striking corymbs of bright orange flowers, and alternate sessile, lanceolate, dark leaves; the root is obtained in grey-white pieces composed of easily separated concentric rings of tissue; the taste is nutty.

Habitat: north-east and south-east North America, Arizona and northern Mexico.

Constituents: glycosides (including asclepiadin and possibly cardioactive glycosides), essential oil.

Actions: relaxing expectorant; diffusive peripheral vasodilator; soothing and diffusing inflammatory lesions, especially in the respiratory system.

Applications: to pulmonary and bronchial infections and congestion (generally combined with ginger or other 'hot' remedy); as a constituent of a fever management regime when of a pulmonary origin.

Dosage: 0.5-3 grams of dried root equivalent three times per day.

---

pneumonia, infection that has spread beyond the bronchial airways to affect the pulmonary tissue itself, marked by often serious impairment of breathing and occasionally fatal febrile response. In three forms: bacterial and viral pneumonia, and bronchopneumonia. The first is the most serious but is much less common nowadays as a result of antibiotic treatment; the last two are for different reasons not so certain to respond to allopathic drug treatment and there is usually scope for conservative therapy, provided of course that the best possible expertise is available. Pneumonia should be suspected in any case of sudden or long-term fever, with hacking cough, blood-flecked, pus-containing or dry mucus, breathlessness, pale or bluish face. Bacterial pneumonia is the most abrupt and severe in symptoms; viral pneumonia is generally of lesser severity and with drier cough; bronchopneumonia is associated with acute **bronchitis,** and tends to have a fluctuating pattern of fever. Herbal therapy will be based on a **fever management** regime with the incorporation as appropriate of such expectorants as thyme, lobelia, garlic, ginger, squill and ipecacuanha. Anti-infective remedies like echinacea will usually be indicated. Specific breathing exercises will need to be invoked and a very long **convalescence** insisted on to prevent secondary complications. It is important to re-emphasize that the use of antibiotics does have an important role to play in saving life in cases of pneumonia and that their use should therefore be well considered.

---

poke root, Coakum, Pigeon berry, Red plant, Pocan, *Phytolacca americana* L., *P. decandra* L. Fam: Phytolaccaceae.
The root of a striking perennial plant up to 4 metres in height (though generally around 1.5-2) with vigorous green or purple stems bearing alternate simple leaves and numerous small white or pale-green flowers in drooping racemes that give way to the clusters of staining purple berries; the root is externally banded with bars of cork, pale yellow-brown in colour, internally paler, and with zones of fibrous elements making it hard to break; the taste is acrid.
Habitat: in damp soils and shady spots in eastern North America, naturalized to southern Europe.
Constituents: triterpenoid saponins (phytolaccosides); alkaloid (phytolaccine), resins, phytolaccic acid, tannin.
Actions: anti-inflammatory, possibly stimulating leucocyte and lymphatic activity.
Applications: to rheumatic and other auto-immune inflammatory conditions; to inflammatory conditions of the respiratory system; to lymphatic swellings and inflammations.
Dosage: 60-300mg of dried root equivalent three times per day.
Caution: in large doses this remedy is an irritant emetic and cathartic; there are also concerns for its wider safety: it would be wise to treat this remedy with considerable respect, and not to use it unless properly trained.

---

poliomyelitis, a viral disease most often affecting the nervous system and thereby sometimes producing atonic paralysis of muscles; most often occurring in children; at least 80-90 per cent of all cases are so mild as to be barely noticed, and are marked only by mild fever, sore throat, malaise, headache, vomiting, these disappearing within 72 hours: sore neck and back and/or muscle tenderness are two features particularly characteristic of the condition and should warn that this is the case. Up to this time treatment can be conservative (*see* **fever management**), but if polio is suspected this should be confirmed and isolation instituted with full medical co-operation; a major priority is *to reduce muscular activity* in the sufferer to a minimum as this is associated with an increased risk of contracting the second stage: cramp bark and other **antispasmodics** and **relaxants** will be useful. Secondary involvement is indicated by a recurrence of fever some days later with stiffness, muscle pain and spasm, and this will demand most expert care to prevent permanent damage. It must be emphasized however, that polio is not an inevitably crippling or killing disease: adequate herbal treatment of the initial attack is likely to further reduce the small chance that the complications will occur. In particular treat all fevers with adequate rest immediately they occur. Even should the paralytic stage develop there is still a relatively small chance that it will become permanent. At all stages therefore positive health and healing measures are well justified.

Polygala senega, snake root.

Polygonum bistorta, bistort.

---

poplar, Quaking aspen, White poplar, *Populus tremuloides* Michx. Fam: Salicaceae.

The dried bark of a slender tree with smooth, light-green bark up to 30 metres in height, with smooth, finely-toothed, pointed ovate leaves; the catkins of staminate flowers are dominated by silky bracts.

Habitat: throughout North America.

Constituents: salicylates (populin, salicin); essential oil (including bisabolol); flavonoids; tannin.

Actions: tonic digestive stimulant; astringent, diuretic.

Applications: to debilitated conditions, especially when marked by looseness of the bowels and digestive inadequacy; for managing digestive and bowel performance in febrile conditions; for associated rheumatic disorders.

Dosage: 1-4 grams of dried bark equivalent three times per day.

Note: the European white poplar or aspen, *P. tremula,* and black poplar *P. nigra* are used for their buds (*see also* **Balm of Gilead**) as expectorant and circulatory stimulant remedies for upper respiratory infections and rheumatic conditions.

Populus gileadensis, Balm of Gilead.

Populus tremuloides, poplar.

---

post-natal depression, an often traumatic emotional lurch after childbirth, largely due to abrupt changes in hormonal levels, particularly the fall in progesterone. Loving support and counselling is vital, but relief may be had with agnus-castus, and with **nervous restoratives** and the **galactogogue** remedies (*see also* **premenstrual tension** for other measures).

Potentilla erecta, tormentil.

---

poultice, a hot pack applied to the skin, often over a wound or other damage, made up by mixing hot water with chopped or ground herbs in a muslin bag; often used to draw pus and other debris from a wound; linseed and comfrey are particularly suited to this technique.

---

pregnancy, a time when the use of herbal remedies needs to be strictly controlled, especially in the first three months. Many herbs have actions on the pregnant uterus (*see also* **abortifacient**), including therapeutic doses of many kitchen herbs like sage, marjoram and parsley, although the tiny amounts used in cooking are safe enough. Other notable examples are juniper, pennyroyal and celery seed, but the best policy is to consider all remedies risky unless reliably informed otherwise. *See also* **morning sickness, labour.**

---

premenstrual tension, symptoms ranging from mild discomfort to serious metabolic, emotional and psychological disruption, with water retention a particularly frequent feature; many other medical conditions are likely to be made worse as well. Due among other factors to a too rapid fall in progesterone levels in relation to oestrogen (and similar in this sense to post-natal depression), and thus associated with a premature cessation of corpus luteum function. The herbal remedy agnus-castus is almost specific, but improvements are also likely with helonias root, dong'quai and parsley. Vitamin B6 and the essential oil of evening primrose have been used with success. **Diuretic** herbs and a low-salt diet may alleviate water retention problems.

---

prickly ash, Toothache bush, *Zanthoxylum americanum* Mill., and *Z. clavaherculis* L. Fam: Rutaceae.
    The bark and berries of a small tree with pinnate leaves and branches covered with strong prickles; the berries grow in clusters at the end of the

branches and are black capsules containing one or two dark seeds; the bark occurs in curved or quilled pieces, externally roughened with patches, furrows and lenticels and occasional spines, with yellowish inner surface with fine longitudinal striations and covered with glistening crystals; the taste of both is bitter and acrid.

Constituents: the bark contains alkaloids (including chelerythrine, magnoflorine, nitidine and lauroflorine).

Actions: stimulant to peripheral circulation (berries slightly more so than the bark); locally counter-irritant.

Applications: to skin, joint and other chronic inflammatory disorders marked by deficient circulation; to cramps and peripheral circulatory disorders.

Dosage: 0.5-3 grams of dried root and 0.5-1.5 grams of dried berries equivalent three times per day.

Primula veris et officinalis,   cowslip.

---

prostate disease,   generally one or more of three distinct types: (1) Prostatis — infection of the prostate gland from either **urinary infection** or **venereal** disease (especially gonorrhoea) or from blood-borne infection; either acute or chronic, with pain or discomfort on passing urine, deep aching in the pelvis and groin, and occasionally fever. Intensive conventional medical treatment may be necessary in a few cases, and in all, only qualified practitioners should be sought; herbal treatment may involve a choice between **urinary antiseptics,** and systemic **alteratives, anti-infectives,** etc., as well as such specific remedies as horsetail, eryngo and gravel-root. (2) Benign prostatic enlargement — an extremely common, even universal feature of aging, but affecting a few particularly badly; symptoms of urinary retention, incontinence, dribbling or reduced flow, urgency, and getting up in the night are common features of the condition; background factors are likely to be a too-rapid fall in testosterone levels in relation to oestrogen, a fall that may be reduced by retaining an active competitive life-style into retirement; specific herbal remedies to reduce the problem include saw palmetto, damiana, horsetail and couch grass, but wider health considerations will usually play an important part. (3) Prostate cancer — a small proportion of enlarged prostates, generally marked by the speed of onset of the symptoms of enlargement, plus increasing pain in the lower back and pelvis. Any treatment can only be attempted after exhaustive discussion and investigation of the individual condition.

Prunus serotina, wild cherry bark.

---

pruritus, or itching is an often distressing accompaniment to inflammation, especially in eczema, anal and vaginal irritation. It is always a priority to correct, as far as possible, underlying causes (like **eczema, vaginal problems, nettle rash, haemorrhoids, chilblains, shingles**). It may be that the itching is caused by contact with irritant material and this should be withdrawn. Other causes are the bites of insects, the presence of pests, scabies, lice and **worms**. Itching may result from **liver disease, diabetes mellitus, kidney diseases,** and a wide range of other systemic conditions. It may accompany pregnancy and the **menopause**. It is often more noticeable in those of a nervous or anxious disposition and **relaxants** may be applicable. It may signify an **allergy** and will often respond to internal administration of **bitter** herbs. It may simply indicate an excessively dry skin, especially in the elderly. For these especially and for all others symptomatic relief may be had with almond and avocado oils, and **demulcent** herbs: chickweed is almost specific for the task.

---

psoriasis, a particularly complex inflammatory disease of the skin, an example of an **auto-immune** disease, to be treated as such; in other words, a search is made for any source of toxicity anywhere in the body, and liver function in particular is reviewed; once such possibilities are explored the use of **alteratives** may be as valuable as in other skin diseases, but Oregon grape, sarsaparilla, burdock root, curled dock and red clover are favoured.

---

psychological problems, *see* **nervous problems.**

---

psyllium, (a) Dark psyllium, Flea seeds, *Plantago psyllium* L. or (b) Pale psyllium, Ispaghula, Spogel seeds, *P. ovata* Forsk. Fam: Plantaginaceae.
The seeds of two species of plantain (a) glossy dark brown to black, often with a reddish hue, 2-3mm long and 0.8-1.2mm wide, oblong with a translucent outer coat revealing the endosperm within; (b) pale grey to pinkish brown, 1-3.5mm long, 1-1.7mm wide, boat-shaped, with a red-brown spot on the convex surface, and a white area on the concave surface marking the hilum; the taste of both is mucilaginous.
Habitat: (a) southern Europe, North Africa and Asia; (b) India and Iran, and cultivated in Spain.
Constituents: mainly mucilage, plus fixed oil.

Actions: bulk laxative; demulcent and healing.

Applications: to sluggish or irritable bowels, helping to regulate movements whatever the dysfunction; as a useful management treatment in bowel disease; locally for infections and furunculosis.

Dosage: 3-10 grams of dried seeds once or twice a day.

---

purgative, a remedy with drastic laxative action, used in traditional practice as an abrupt method of emptying the gut contents and increasing the elimination raté of bile; generally used along with **emetic** remedies; like the latter only appropriate for those of very robust constitution and not applied in modern practice very often. Most purgative remedies are now considered too toxic for everyday use: examples are jalap, bitter apple and scammony. *See* **laxative** and **aperient** for less drastic techniques.

---

pyelonephritis, or pyelitis, is infection of the kidney, most often arising from previous **urinary infection,** but also possibly due to blood-borne infection from septic tonsils, throat, gums, or boils or abscesses elsewhere. Can be acute or chronic, is usually accompanied by fever, pain in the loins, frequency of urination with scalding pain and scanty flow. Treatment will combine conservative measures and **fever management** where appropriate, and treatment of whatever cause is apparent, e.g., with **urinary antiseptics, anti-infective** or **antiseptic** remedies. It must be conducted only by qualified practitioners, and referral to a doctor or hospital may have to be considered.

Pyrethrum parthenium, feverfew.

Q

---

quassia, Bitter wood, *Picrasma excelsa* (Sw) Planch., *Picraena excelsa* Lindl. Fam: Simarubaceae.

The wood of a tall tree obtained as fibrous pale-yellow chips with an intense bitter taste.

Habitat: the West Indies and especially Jamaica.

Constituents: bitter glycosides ('quassiin': including picrasmin, quassin); alkaloid.

Applications: to debilitated digestion and loss of appetite, as in convalescence or cachexia; to nematode infestations.

Dosage: 0.3-0.6 gram of dried wood equivalent three times per day.

---

quebracho, White quebracho, *Aspidosperma quebracho-blanco* Schlecht. Fam: Apocynaceae.

The bark of a tall evergreen tree obtained in very thick pieces covered with a thick, fissured and furrowed greyish cork layer with a yellowish-brown striated fibrous inner layer; the taste is very bitter.

Habitat: South America.

Constituents: indole alkaloids (including aspidospermine, quebrachamine, quebrachine).

Actions: bronchial relaxant and antispasmodic; respiratory stimulant; peripheral vasodilator; bitter digestive tonic.

Applications: taken tonically to relieve asthmatic and other conditions of bronchial constriction; traditionally used in fever management, particularly with respiratory involvement.

Dosage: the maximum permitted dose is 50mg, the recommended initial dose being about 30mg of dried bark equivalent three times per day.

Caution: large doses of this remedy are emetic and cathartic and it is restricted in the U.K. to practitioners only.

---

queen's delight, Yaw root, *Stillingia sylvatica* L. Fam: Euphorbiaceae.

The root of a perennial herb up to 1.5 metres high with alternate leathery, sessile leaves and a terminal spike of yellow flowers, exuding an acrid milky juice when cut; the root is obtained chopped into pieces, externally red-brown thick cork, internally pale pink-brown, the wood fibrous; the taste is acrid and bitter.

Habitat: acid and sandy soils of southern United States.

Constituents: acrid resin and fixed oil, volatile oil, tannin.

Action: circulatory stimulant and diaphoretic; in low doses stimulating expectorant and laxative (in high doses irritant emetic and cathartic); stimulating alterative.

Applications: to chronic exudative skin diseases; to bronchitic congestion.

Dosage: 0.5-2 grams of dried root equivalent three times per day.

Caution: this remedy is always irritating to the mucous membranes and must be used with care, never in large doses or after storage of more than two years.

Quercus robur,   oak bark.

---

quinsy,   an abscess associated with the tonsils, *see* **tonsillitis.**

R

Ranunculus ficaria,   pilewort.

---

raspberry,   *Rubus idaeus* L. Fam: Rosaceae.
    The leaves of a perennial herb with creeping rootstock and biennial, slightly prickly, flowering stems up to 1.5 metres high; the leaves are divided into three to five pointed and toothed leaflets, light green above and whitish underneath; long panicles of white flowers with short, narrow petals giving way to the familiar red fruit.
    Habitat: in woods throughout Britain, Europe and northern Asia.
    Constituents: tannins, other poorly determined principles.
    Actions: toning the gravid uterus; locally astringent.
    Applications: to easing and improving the efficiency of labour, taken increasingly through the last three months of pregnancy; mouth and throat inflammations and infections as a mouthwash and gargle; as an eye lotion for conjunctival problems.
    Dosage: 2-8 grams of the dried leaf in infusion three times per day.

Note: the wild North American raspberry *Rubus strigosus* may be used instead of *R. idaeus.*

Raynaud's disease,   a condition of excessive constriction of the peripheral blood vessels leading to severe whitening and numbing of the fingers and even hands, occasionally toes and nose; there is often a tendency for circulation to return dramatically and painfully. The condition may arise from **auto-immune** or **allergy** diseases, or may be linked with other systemic problems: such possibilities must be thoroughly explored in treatment, but for relief of the symptoms, **circulatory stimulants** and **peripheral vasodilators** are effective. Smoking, alchohol and caffeine are exacerbatory in most cases; where nervous tension or anxiety are factors the use of cramp bark and other **anti-spasmodics** may be extremely useful.

---

red clover, Purple clover, Trefoil, *Trifolium pratense* L. Fam: Papilionaceae.

The flowerheads of a biennial or perennial plant up to 60cm in height with globular red-to-purple flowerheads subtended by a pair of trifoliate sessile leaves.

Habitat: widespread in grassy spaces throughout the world, generally as an introduction.

Constituents: phenolic glycosides, flavonoids, cyanogenic glycosides, coumarins.

Actions: an alterative remedy; diuretic; expectorant; possibly oestrogenic.

Applications: to toxic conditions such as skin disease; has been used in the herbal treatment of cancer, especially of the breast and ovaries.

Dosage: 3-6 grams of the dried flower equivalent three times per day.

---

relaxants, herbal remedies that appear to relax the whole body, not only mentally, but particularly in terms of visceral neuromuscular function (they may often be described as relaxing 'from the neck down' to differentiate them from tranquillizers.) The term is preferred here to the traditional **'antispasmodic',** as it emphasizes their overall calming action. Relaxants are indicated whenever it is desired to reduce the effect of tension or constitutional overactivity on a body function; they are, for instance, ideal for supporting recovery in illnesses of children when their innate excitability and restlessness is the main obstacle to calm progress, and this obvious example can be extended to illustrate the application of relaxants to adults; in practice relaxants will be used to give the body the opportunity of finding a healthy balance in such cases as nervous **dyspepsia, nervous bowel, constipation** of tense origin, bronchial spasm, vascular spasm, spasmodic **dysmenorrhoea,** certain cases of **migraine,** and any other visceral, physiological or even organic disorder where tissue tension can be elicited (tension in this sense is often synonymous with overactivity). In short relaxant remedies provide an important tool in managing disease conditions: most are wholly safe and non-addictive (many are actually so gentle that their effect is built up only gradually), and above all they do not depress vital recuperative functions; they are thus an ideal accompaniment for **circulatory stimulants** and digestive and other stimulating or tonifying treatments, allowing restoration to proceed without the distractions and debilitating effects of tension or overactivity. They are a very important herbal strategy. A list of relaxant herbs would include chamomile, lemon balm, limeflowers, lavender, lobelia, vervain, rosemary, St John's wort, catmint, betony, (American) ginseng, motherwort, pasque flower, valerian, scullcap, passionflower, golden rod, both horehounds, mistletoe and wild yam. *See also* **sedative** *and* **nervous problems** for more purely nervous orientation.

---

resins,   hard brittle secretions from certain plants that soften on heating; they are very complex chemically; they are likely to play a significant part in the action of several herbal remedies, probably acting to stimulate white blood cell activity near contacted mucous surfaces; however, such activity is only likely in alcoholic tinctures or chloroform solutions of the relevant herbs as resins are quite insoluble in water; key resin-containing herbs include myrrh, marigold, balm of Gilead, kava-kava, lignum vitae and hops.

Rhamnus frangula,   alder buckthorn.

Rhamnus purshiana,   cascara sagrada.

---

rhatany root,   Peruvian rhatany, *Krameria triandra* Ruiz and Pavon. Fam: Krameriaceae.
    The root of a low shrub with year-long red flowers on procumbent stems; the root is obtained in large or small fragments, dark red-brown externally, scaly and rough when old, smooth but fissured on the young roots; the bark is very fibrous and relatively thick, the inner wood is pale red-brown, porous and splintery; the bark tastes astringent.
    Habitat: dry, gravelly slopes of Peru and Bolivia.
    Constituents: condensed and hydrolysable tannins; krameric acid.
    Actions: astringent and styptic.
    Applications: to local application, to bleeding and discharging mucosal

or epithelial surfaces, haemorrhoids, chilblains, etc.; to manage diarrhoea.
Dosage: 0.5-2 grams of dried root equivalent three times per day.

---

rheumatic fever, an acute form of rheumatism found mostly in children, heralded by sore throat followed 1-3 weeks later by fever with transient joint pains, and occasionally muscular spasms (chorea or St Vitus's dance); it appears to be an overreaction in certain dispositions to streptococcal infections; it should not be treated by unqualified practitioners due to the risk of inflammatory damage to the heart, of severe, possibly fatal, rises in body temperature, and of lung disease. Qualified practitioners may, subject to the need for conventional drug treatment, manage the fever with appropriate remedies (*see* **fever management**), relieving the often very painful joints with wintergreen oil, and relying more than usually on **anti-infective** remedies, especially garlic and echinacea; adrenal cortex function has been shown to be constitutionally weak in sufferers and licorice may be indicated. After acute attacks there should be at least a week's bed rest to avoid further heart complications. **Eliminative** and **anti-infective** remedies may be used as indicated as part of a regime of **convalescence** to reduce the likely risk of re-occurrence.

---

rheumatism, muscular, *see* **myalgia.**

---

rheumatoid arthritis, an inflammatory disease of the joints, a classic example of an **auto-immune disease,** where the joint tissues are attacked by the body's own defences; may be associated in the early stages with a fever, but most often seen as a shifting attack on one or more joints at a time, not specifically those under most strain (*see* **osteoarthritis**), often settling on the fingers but sometimes involving many joints in increasing pain, swelling and immobility. Primary herbal treatment is to reduce any toxic exacerbation, as with other auto-immune conditions: it has been conclusively shown that patients are much more likely to have had serious lung diseases in the past, or be prone to low-grade problems currently, or smoke; thus suitable **expectorants** may be indicated to cleanse the lung of accumulations; similar attention may be paid to the urinary system and **urinary antiseptics** used if indicated; the throat, liver and digestive tract in general are all liable sources of exacerbation, appropriate cleansing of which can significantly improve the rheumatic condition. Specific **anti-inflammatory** remedies may be used both locally and systemically, to alleviate the condition while background factors are investigated, and the following herbs may be of particular benefit: lignum-vitae, arbor-vitae, buckbean, black cohosh, devil's claw, sarsaparilla, gotu kola and wild yam. The possibility of **food allergies** must be investigated. As the disease is much more predominant in women, it is often profitable to check on hormonal factors (*see* **hormonal remedies**). Dietary precautions as appropriate for **arthritis** in general should always be instituted.

---

ribwort, English plantain, Ribwort, Plantain, Ribgrass, Jackstraw, *Plantago lanceolata* L. Fam: Plantaginaceae.

The leaves of a common member of the plantain family, these rising as a rosette from a short, thick, multi-branched rootstock, each leaf 5-25cm long with three to five prominent longitudinal ribs; the flowerstalks, longer than the leaves, support the characteristic elongated or round flowerhead, greenish at first but turning black-brown on ripening.

Habitat: very common on pastures, roadsides, banks, wasteplaces, preferring dry sandy soil, throughout Britain and all the temperate world.

Constituents: mucilage, glycosides (including aucubin), tannins, silica, zinc and high levels of potassium.

Actions: soothing and healing locally; taken internally a relaxing **expectorant,** toning the respiratory mucous membranes and checking excessive catarrh; calming urinary spasm and pains.

Applications: to bronchial spasm, nervous and dry coughing, allergic and other cases of rhinitis, nasal and middle ear catarrhal conditions; painful and irritating urinary conditions as at least a short-term palliative; for the restoration of lungs after serious pulmonary diseases; locally as a wound healer.

Dosage: 1-4 grams of dried leaf equivalent three or more times a day.

---

ringworm, and other fungal infections of the skin or nails may be treated locally with anti-fungal tinctures such as marigold, arbor-vitae and myrrh, and systemically with **anti-infective, eliminative** and **alterative** remedies. Poke root is particularly likely to be effective.

Rosa canina, rose-hips.

---

rosacea, *see* **acne rosacea.**

---

rose-hips, Dog-rose, Brier rose, *Rosa canina* L. Fam: Rosaceae.

The fruit of an erect or straggling woody shrub, the woody stems giving rise to weak, branched flowering shoots of up to 3 metres in length with curved prickles; the leaves are divided into five to seven toothed leaflets; single or small groups of white or pink sweet-scented flowers found at the shoot tips, give way to the ovoid or globular fruit.

Habitat: abundant in hedges and thickets throughout Britain, Europe and northern Asia, also naturalized on the east coast of North America.

Constituents: ascorbic acid, flavonoids, fruit acids, tannin, mucilage, provitamin A.

Actions: dietary supplement; astringent.

Applications: to supplementing vitamin C levels; for mild infections, particularly of the respiratory system, and for the common cold; for gastric inflammations and enteritis with diarrhoea.

Dosage: 2-10 grams of dried hips equivalent as fresh hip syrup three times per day.

Rosmarinus officinalis, rosemary.

---

rosemary, *Rosmarinus officinalis* L. Fam: Labiatae.

A familiar shrub with narrow, linear, revolute leaves and pale-blue labiate flowers and a strong aromatic, almost camphoraceous odour.

Habitat: indigenous to southern Europe but widely cultivated elsewhere.

Constituents: volatile oil (including borneol, linalool, pinene, camphene, cineol, camphor); tannins; bitter principle; resin.

Actions: stimulant to peripheral circulation and diaphoretic; relaxant, antispasmodic and restorative to the nervous system; reputed cardiac tonic, cholagogue.

Applications: depression and debility linked to nervous tension; vasoconstrictory headaches and migraines (those improving with heat, *see* **feverfew**); to palpitations and other signs of nervous tension affecting the circulation; dyspeptic conditions with flatulence and signs of liver inadequacy; any condition where poor circulation and liver function are combined; locally as a wash for dandruff and scurf.

Dosage: 1-4 grams of dried herb equivalent three times per day.

---

rubefacient, a term used to describe an agent that when applied to the skin produces a local vasodilation in the underlying tissues (indicated as a reddening of the skin); the actual effect can range from a mild flush right through to blistering (*see* **vesicant**). The principle behind the application of rubefacients is that the increased blood flow will improve the cleansing and nourishing of the affected tissues; in particular the aim is to aid the processes of **inflammation** in resolving and cleansing damaged or toxic tissues.

Rubefacients are thus sometimes referred to as 'counter-irritants' for their effect in stimulating an extra 'therapeutic' inflammatory response; unlike the normal inflammation there is little of histamine and other pain-inducing agents released, so the beneficial effect is obtained without complications. The technique is applied particularly to arthritic joints, but may also help in pleurisy and other relatively superficial inflammations. Many **circulatory stimulants** are rubefacient, notably the 'hot spices' like cayenne, the mustards, horscradish, ginger and others such as kava-kava and prickly ash. Their use is best left to qualified practitioners; however the familiar mustard bath for hands and feet, using a weak solution of mustard powder in hot water, is a surprisingly rewarding regular treatment for arthritic and rheumatic problems in those areas.

Rubus fructicosus, blackberry.

Rubus idaeus, raspberry.

rue, Herb-of-grace, Herby grass, *Ruta graveolens* L. Fam: Rutaceae.
A perennial herb or shrub with alternate tri- or bipinnate leaves and terminal panicles of yellowish-green flowers; the whole plant has a strong unpleasant odour and a bitter and acrid taste.

Habitat: indigenous to southern Europe but widely cultivated elsewhere.

Constituents: volatile oil (including methyl and nonyl ketones); flavonoids (notably rutin); furanocoumarins (including bergapten, rutarellin, xanthotoxin); alkaloids (including skimmiarin and possibly some of the berberine group), tannins.

Actions: circulatory stimulant; uterine stimulant; antispasmodic; stimulating expectorant (emetic in even moderate doses).

Applications: to bronchial and croupy conditions; to amenorrhoea where pregnancy has been positively excluded.

Dosage: 0.2-1 gram of dried herb equivalent three times a day (before meals).

Caution: this remedy must not be used in pregnancy; it has emetic tendencies and low doses are strongly advisable.

Rumex crispus,　curled dock.

Ruta graveolens,　rue.

S

Sabal serrulatum,　saw palmetto.

sage,　Red sage, *Salvia officinalis* L. Fam: Labiatae.
The leaves of a shrubby herb; hairy, leathery greyish-green or purplish-red, with reticulated veins; the purple labiate flowers grow in whorls in the upper stems; the whole herb has a characteristic taste and odour.
Habitat: indigenous to southern Europe but widely cultivated all over the world.
Constituents: volatile oil (including thujone, linalool, borneol, camphor, salvene, pinene and many others); oestrogenic substances; triterpenoid saponins; flavonoids; tannins; resin.
Actions: astringent, healing and antiseptic on mucosal surfaces; peripheral vasodilator but suppressing perspiration; reduces salivation and lactation; uterine stimulant; cholagogue.
Applications: as a mouthwash and gargle to affections of the throat and mouth; to restore digestive and circulatory function in debility and convalescence; to night sweats and excessive perspiration or salivation; to soothing and regulating hormonal problems in menopause.
Dosage: 0.5-3 grams of dried leaves three times per day.
Caution: this remedy should be used carefully and avoided altogether in pregnancy.

St John's wort,　*Hypericum perforatum,* L. Fam: Hypericaceae.
An erect perennial herb about 0.5m in height, with bright-yellow five-petalled flowers at the end of multi-branched smooth stems; when held to the light the small oblong leaves are seen to possess tiny perforations.

Habitat: throughout Britain, Europe and Asia, as well as North America, on roadsides and banks, and in woods and hedgerows, preferring open situations and dry soils.

Constituents: glycosides (including a red pigment, hypericin); flavonoids; tannins; resin; and a volatile oil.

Action: the herb has gentle calming effect when taken internally, this conveniently combining with a restorative tonic effect on the nervous system; the red oil made by standing the flowers in oil in sunlight for two weeks has local analgesic and slightly antiseptic effects. The whole plant is astringent and promotes healing.

Applications: Internally for anxiety states, tension and irritability, particularly where these have persisted long enough to lead to fatigue or depression. The red oil is used externally on unbroken skin for light burns, neuralgia and fibrositis; the whole herb makes a good external wound application.

Dosage: 1-4 grams dried herb equivalent three times per day.

Salix alba et spp,   willow bark.

---

salpingitis,   *see* **pelvic infection.**

Salvia officinalis,   sage.

Sambucus nigra,   elder.

Sanguinaria canadensis,   blood root.

Sanguisorba officinalis,   burnet, greater.

---

saponins,   complex glycosides found in many plants, marked by their soapy quality in watery solution (e.g., they form a lather when dissolved and shaken: a simple way of judging whether a plant contains saponins); until relatively recently their main effect on the body was judged in terms of their local detergent effect on the gut wall (many are stimulating **expectorants,** or **emetics** in quantity), with fears, generally unfounded, for their wider toxicity (they must never be injected into the body, but digestion breaks down their detergent effect before it can do harm internally). In recent years, however, notably in relation to Asiatic ginseng and similar plants, the hormonal changes effected by the saponins have become obvious: saponins have a steroidal structure similar to steroidal hormones like the stress and sex hormones produced by the adrenal cortex and gonads respectively; it appears that, in some plants at least, the saponins have the ability to regulate the switching mechanisms that regulate steroidal hormone activity within the body. Some are thus thought to account for the activity of those remedies that are hormonal **adaptogens,** and others have known effects on the endocrine system. In Chinese medicine, many of the most respected 'king' remedies, used effectively as adaptogens, are saponin-containing. Notable examples in the present text are the ginsengs, licorice, helonias root, blue cohosh, squaw vine, wild yam and fenugreek. Expectorant herbs with saponin content include squills, cowslip, mullein flowers, violet, heartsease, snakeroot and licorice. Some saponins actually settle digestion as in those of asparagus, oats and many vegetables; others appear to contribute **diuretic** effects (as in birch and corn silk), **anti-inflammatory** action (as in figwort, sarsaparilla, licorice, wild yam and the ginsengs), and a few appear to exert an interesting effect on blood vessel walls (those of horse chestnut, limeflowers and yarrow).

Sarothamnus scoparius, broom.

---

sarsaparilla, *Smilax spp.* Fam: Liliaceae.
The root of various species of perennial climbers obtained commercially as long, slender, red to orange-brown rootlets with pale cortex and fibrous yellow core; the taste is slightly acrid and bitter and there is no odour.
Habitat: Jamaica, Honduras, Costa Rica, Mexico.
Constituents: steroidal saponins (including sarsaponin, parillin); sterols; essential oil; resin.
Actions: alterative; gentle circulatory stimulant; slightly testosteronal.
Applications: to rheumatic and psoriatic and other chronic inflammatory diseases.
Dosage: 1-4 grams of dried root equivalent three times per day.

---

sassafras, Cinnamon wood, Ague tree, *Sassafras albidum* (Nutt) Nees.
Fam: Lucraceae.
The root and bark of a tree up to 12 metres in height with smooth orange-

brown bark and many slender branches, variable green or reddish foliage and small insignificant flowers; it is obtained in irregular pieces of curved or quilled root bark, reddish-brown in colour, the inner surface darker than the outer, the outer surface grey and rough where the cork is present; the odour is strongly fragrant, the taste is sweet and aromatic.

Habitat: in deciduous woodland in eastern North America.

Constituents: volatile oil (including mainly safrole), condensed tannins, resin, cinnamic acid derivatives.

Actions: alterative; warming peripheral vasodilator with apparently a specific cleansing action on the cutaneous tissues; carminative; diuretic.

Applications: to eruptive and inflamed skin diseases (generally combined with other alterative agents).

Dosage: 1-3 grams of dried root bark equivalent three times per day.

Caution: the constituent of the volatile oil, safrole, is both neuro- and hepatotoxic; this is very unlikely to be a factor in using the remedy in normal therapeutic dosages, but Oil of Sassafras is still sometimes obtainable and this should never be used internally (it is traditionally used locally for scabies and other infestations).

Sassafras albidum, sassafras.

---

saw palmetto, Sabal, *Serenoa serrulata* Hook., *S. repens* Bartram., *Sabal serrulatum* Roem & Schult. Fam: Palmae.

The berries of a low scrubby palm with a largely subterranean trunk; above the ground this is covered with the bases of withered leaves, although these may remain as twiggy, prostrate branches; the stiff leaves, 60cm long grow in fans; clusters of ivory-white fragrant flowers are formed and these give way to 2cm-long stone fruits, dark-purple to black, with light brown flesh; the odour is very pungent.

Habitat: on sand dunes and coastal regions of Florida, Texas and Georgia.

Constituents: volatile oil, steroidal saponins, resins, tannins, fixed oil, possible alkaloid.

Actions: toning the male reproductive system and particularly the prostate; urinary antiseptic; acting to reduce congestive catarrhal conditions of the respiratory system; relaxant.

Applications: to prostatic hypertrophy and other prostatic ailments; to debilitated conditions of the male reproductive system; to male senility and wider debility; to urinary infections; for respiratory catarrh in the above circumstances.

Dosage: 1-2 grams of dried berry pulp equivalent three times per day.

---

scarlet fever, essentially an acute streptoccocal infection of the throat, now rarely as severe in developed countries as formerly; manifested as sore throat with fever, often with vomiting, a transient rash of tiny spots over the body; treatment can be conservative (*see* **fever management** *and* **throat problems**), but secondary complications are possible (e.g., **rheumatic fever** a fortnight later, nephritis and middle ear infection, *see* **ear problems**) and must be guarded against, possibly with the use of **anti-infective** remedies.

---

schizophrenia, *see* **nervous problems.**

---

sciatica, a painful condition of the sciatic nerve running down the leg generally due to pressure on it as it passes through the lower spine and pelvis. Primary concern is to relieve the pelvic condition, most often a 'slipped disc', by rest, proper lumbar support and possibly manipulation by osteopath or chiropractor. Contributory muscle tension may be relieved with herbal **relaxants** and there may be scope for treating the condition as a nerve inflammation (*see* **neuralgia**).

Scolopendrium vulgare, Hart's-tongue fern.

Scrophularia nodosa, figwort.

---

scullcap, Skullcap, Mad-dog weed, Blue scullcap, Helmet flower, *Scutellaria laterifolia* L. Fam: Labiatae.

A perennial plant up to a metre in height with opposite, serrated ovate leaves and one-sided racemes of characteristic pale-blue flowers. Two-lipped with the upper in the shape of a helmet, the calyx surviving to cover the seeds; notoriously difficult to obtain in pure unsubstituted form in the U.K.: best to assume that any given sample is *not* scullcap unless good evidence to the contrary.

Habitat: wet ground of north-eastern North America.

Constituents: flavonoid glycosides (including scutellarin and scutellarein), bitter, volatile oil.

Actions: central nervous relaxant and restorative; antispasmodic.

Applications: to nervous tension; to neurological and neuromotor conditions, including epilepsy, helping to reduce the severity and frequency of symptoms; to states of nervous exhaustion and debility.
Dosage: 0.5-2 grams of dried herb equivalent three times per day.

Note: the common scullcap, *S. galericulata* L. of northern temperate zones around the globe (including Britain and Europe), has recently been used as a substitute with many of the effects of *S. laterifolia.*

Scutellaria laterifolia, scullcap.

---

sea holly, *see* **eryngo.**

---

sedative, a term used to define a remedy that induces a reduction in nervous activity; it is applied mostly to those remedies which are used to reduce nervous tension, pain and neuromuscular spasm (but *see also* **relaxant, analgesic**) and to help induce sleep (*see* **insomnia**). By definition, sedatives are to varying degrees depressant agents, and their use should be minimized (in Galenic terms the sedatives were considered 'cold' in character, the stronger the sedative, the 'colder', i.e., nearer death, it was). In any positive approach to health the sedative is seen at best as a necessary evil, having at most the potential of freeing the body from the disabling effects of pain and tension, possibly allowing rest and the sparks of recovery to be generated: but they are always seen as depressing vitality. The most widespread herbal sedative in traditional times was the opium poppy, still the source of the morphine and codeine group of drugs; the modern herbalist will consider the use of remedies of lesser impact, examples being wild lettuce, yellow jasmine, Jamaican dogwood, wild cherry, cowslip, lady's slipper, hops, jimson weed, henbane and deadly nightshade. It must be said, however, that the use of any of this group must be carefully considered, and preferably left to a qualified practitioner; several of the remedies are dangerous enough to be legally unavailable to anyone else. *See also* **relaxant** for a more positive approach to tension.

Senecio aureus, life root.

---

senna, (a) Alexandrian senna, *Cassia senna* L., or *C. acutifolia* Delile.,

(b) Tinnevelly senna, *C. angustifolia* Vahl. Fam: Leguminosae.

The fruits ('pods') and leaves of two species of shrub with pinnate leaves in four to five pairs of narrow lanceolate leathery leaflets; yellow flowers are produced at stem tips, giving way to flat oblong seed pods about 4-5cm long, each containing about six seeds; the taste is only slightly bitter, and there is little odour.

Habitat: (a) Sudan and southern Egypt; (b) Saudi Arabia, but also cultivated in southern India.

Constituents: anthraquinones (including rhein, aloe-emodin, sennosides A & B); flavonoids; resin; tartaric acid; mucilage; traces of tannin.

Actions: stimulating laxative.

Applications: to flaccid or atonic constipation, preferably only for short periods.

Dosage: 0.5-2 grams of dried pods or leaves equivalent before retiring (usually taken in warm infusion: 3-6 pods of Alexandrian and 4-12 pods of Tinnevelly).

Caution: not recommended for tense or spastic constipation (see constipation); to prevent griping, carminatives such as fennel or dill may be used.

Serenoa serrulata et spp,   saw palmetto.

---

serpyllum,   *see* **thyme, wild.**

---

seven barks,   Hydrangea, Wild Hydrangea, *Hydrangea arborescens* L. Fam: Saxifragaceae.

The rhizome and roots of a shrub up to 3 metres in height, the stems of which are covered with thin layers of multicoloured bark; there are opposite, ovate, serrate leaves and clusters of small creamy flowers; the rhizome is obtained in pale-yellow woody chips with fragments of thin brown cork, along with short pieces of thin, fibrous roots.

Habitat: woodland and stream banks of south-eastern and central North America.

Constituents: glycoside (hydrangin), saponins, resins.

Actions: diuretic.

Applications: to urinary calculi, urinary infections and prostatitis.

Dosage: 1-4 grams of dried rhizome and roots equivalent three times per day.

---

shepherd's purse, *Capsella bursa-pastoris* L. Fam: Cruciferae.

A small erect herb with a long tapering root supporting a rosette of dentate leaves from the centre of which a stem arises to 15-50cm high; at the top are the small white flowers that give way as the stem grows further to the characteristic purse-shaped fruits densely packed with seeds; the taste is acrid.

Habitat: an extremely common weed of cultivation all over the world; probably originating in southern Europe or western Asia.

Constituents: saponins, mustard oils, flavonoids, resin, monoamines, choline.

Actions: anti-haemorrhagic; urinary antiseptic; circulatory stimulant.

Applications: to excessive menstrual bleeding; nose-bleeds and to help heal the source of blood in the urine (possibly a serious symptom that must be checked); for urinary infections and stones.

Dosage: 1-3 grams of dried herb equivalent three times per day.

---

shingles, or herpes zoster, is an infection of nerve fibres produced by the same virus that causes chickenpox. It is marked by the appearance of clusters of painful blisters where the branches of the affected nerves end, most often on one side of the face, or on the side of the trunk; they most often signal a degree of debility and the herbal approach is to use **nervous restoratives** and other agents to build up strength where appropriate. A persistent **neuralgia** is common after the blisters have gone but this will usually respond to herbs for that condition.

Silybum marianum, milk thistle.

---

sinusitis, inflammation and/or infection of the sinus cavities of the skull, generally secondary to chronic catarrhal conditions of the nasal passages, but occasionally due to dental trouble. Treatment is as for **catarrh,** with special emphasis on steam inhalations and, in most cases, **circulatory stimulants.**

---

skunk cabbage, Meadow cabbage, Polecat weed, *Symplocarpus foetidus* (L) Salisb. Fam: Araceae.

The root and rhizome of a perennial plant with heart-shaped yellow and purple cabbage-like leaves and small spikes of small purplish flowers covered by a spathe the same colour as the leaves; the fleshy rootstock is dark and knotted, with white flesh; the odour is foetid.

Habitat: wet ground and swamps of eastern North America.

Constituents: volatile oil, resin, acrid principle.

Actions: relaxing expectorant; antispasmodic

Applications: to irritable coughs and asthmatic conditions, or other cases where nervous tensions involve the respiratory system.

Dosage: 0.5-1 gram of dried rhizome and roots equivalent three times per day.

---

slippery elm, Red elm, Moose elm, *Ulmus fulva* Michaux. Fam: Ulmaceae.

The inner bark of a small tree with rough branches carrying alternate, irregularly serrated long leaves, rough above and downy below, and dense axillary clusters of small flowers; the leaf buds are covered with a dense yellow wool; the bark is obtained whole or powdered (though the former is now not permitted to be sold in the U.K. because of its traditional use as a mechanical abortifacient): the powder is pale pink-brown in colour with a mucilaginous taste (and character, when mixed with water).

Habitat: eastern and central North America.

Constituents: mucilage, tannin.

Actions: demulcent and emollient; nutritive.

Applications: to irritated mucosa of the oesophagus, stomach and duodenum, having a simple physical soothing action; as a soothing nutritious agent in sensitive digestion during convalescence; locally as a poultice for boils and abscesses.

Dosage: 1-8 grams of dried inner bark powder equivalent (easiest taken in capsules) three times per day before or after meals depending on site of irritation.

Smilax spp, sarsaparilla.

---

snake root, Senega snakeroot, Rattlesnake root, Milkwort, *Polygala senega* L. Fam: Polygalaceae.

The roots of a perennial plant about 30cm high with small, alternate, lanceolate leaves and narrow spikes of small pink-white flowers; the subterranean parts consist of a knotty rootstock with many stem scars and rudimentary purplish leaf buds, with a tortuous taproot and lateral side roots, the whole sinuous and snakelike with a distinct keel line following a spiral course; brown externally, pale yellow inside; the taste is sweet then acrid, producing considerable saliva.

Habitat: rocky and hilly terrain in eastern North America.

Constituents: saponins (including senegin and polygalic acid), salicylates, mucilage, resin.

Actions: irritant to mucous membranes, promoting reflex expectoration, salivation, and in large doses emesis and catharsis; peripheral circulatory stimulant and diaphoretic.

Applications: to chronic bronchitis and bronchial and pulmonary congestions, especially when associated with a sensitivity to the cold.

Dosage: 0.5-1 gram of dried root equivalent three times per day.

Solanum dulcamara, bittersweet.

Solidago virgaurea, golden rod.

---

southernwood, Lads's love, Old man, *Artemisia abrotanum* L. Fam: Compositae.

A shrubby plant with very fine bipinnate leaves with linear pointed segments and a strong characteristic fragrance, and an aromatic bitter taste.

Habitat: indigenous to Spain and Italy but widely cultivated as a garden plant elsewhere.

Constituents: volatile oil with bitter sesquiterpene lactones.

Actions: uterine stimulant; bitter digestive tonic; anthelmintic.

Applications: to reduced menstrual flow; has been used for intestinal worms, especially thread worms.

Dosage: 1-4 grams dried herb equivalent three times per day.

Caution: to be avoided in pregnancy.

---

sprains, healing may be encouraged by external applications or arnica and comfrey.

---

squaw vine, Checkerberry, Partridge berry, *Mitchella repens* L. Fam: Rubiaceae.

A small, prostrate, perennial, evergreen herb with opposite ovate-orbicular leaves and two sessile white flowers at the tip, these giving way to red or occasionally white berries; there is a slightly bitter taste.

Habitat: on woodland floors in eastern North America.

Constituents: saponins, bitter principle, mucilage, tannins.

Actions: nervous tonic and restorative; partus praeparator; uterine relaxant.

Applications: to facilitate labour and delivery in pregnancy; to dysmenorrhoea; to nervous debility, exhaustion or irritability in both sexes, especially when involving symptoms in the reproductive system.

Dosage: 1-4 grams of dried herb equivalent three times per day.

---

squill, *Urginea maritima* (L) Baker. Fam: Liliaceae.

The sliced bulb of an onion-like plant, the bulb consisting of fleshy scaly leaves, the outer ones being reddish or nearly white, half emerging from the ground and giving rise to a smooth, succulent, flowering stem up to 2 metres in height, covered on its upper third with white flowers; the broad lance-shaped leaves follow later; the taste of the bulb is mucilaginous and bitter and it is obtained in curved, straight or triangular slices.

Habitat: dry sandy places in countries bordering the Mediterranean.

Constituents: cardiac glycosides (bufadienolides: scillaren A + B), mucilage, tannin, volatile and fixed oils.

Actions: stimulating expectorant (emetic in large doses); cardioactive; diuretic.

Applications: to chronic and congestive bronchial and pulmonary conditions, notably when associated with symptoms of right-heart difficulty.

Dosage: 60-200mg of dried bulb equivalent three times per day.

Caution: as primarily a gastric irritant this remedy is often poorly accepted unless the dose is low; it is not recommended in acute or active inflammatory states.

Stellaria media, chickweed.

Sticta pulmonaria, lungwort.

Stillingia sylvatica, queen's delight.

---

stimulant, a term meaning different things in different circumstances, but often applied in the context of herbal medicine to those remedies that increase activity in body functions without regard for the inherent capacity of the system to support that activity: in other words they are intrinsically exhausting. This pejorative sense is that applied to caffeine, nicotine, alcohol and other stimulating drugs, but it may also be seen to apply in part to herbal remedies like kola and maté. These latter find application as part of a calculated regime to reassert vitality and activity, but only in consort with **nervous restorative** and other tonifying measures, and for a restricted period. In **physiomedicalism** the term 'stimulant' has been used to describe a remedy that is seen to arouse latent potential for activity; this clearly is a more positive agent in promoting health, and it was a term used for some of their most valuable remedies; thus cayenne was seen as a circulatory stimulant, the **bitters** as digestive stimulants, bayberry as a smooth muscle stimulant and cramp bark as a peripheral nervous stimulant (though acting as a smooth muscle relaxant). Even in this perspective, however, it was considered important to provide adequate restorative back-up whenever there was doubt about the extent of constitutional reserves.

---

stomach problems, *see* **dyspepsia, gastritis, ulcer (peptic)** *and* **hyperacidity.**

---

stone root, Hardback, Knob root, *Collinsonia canadensis* L. Fam: Labiatae.

The rhizome of a perennial herb with greenish-yellow flowers in a loose-panicled raceme; the rhizome is very hard and knobbly, internally yellow and white; the taste is bitter and disagreeably pungent.

Habitat: damp woods throughout eastern North America.

Constituents: saponin, alkaloid, resin, tannin.

Actions: diuretic; gentle peripheral vasodilator and diaphoretic; locally astringent and healing; alterative.

Applications: to urinary calculi; to enteric and bowel disease.

Dosage: 1-4 grams of dried rhizome equivalent three times per day.

---

stroke, a circulatory accident in the brain, either cerebral haemorrhage or cerebral **thrombosis.** Both are associated with age and **arteriosclerosis.** The main priority in treatment is to improve the recovery of those who have already suffered strokes and who may have impaired muscular or speech performance. Useful remedies to take as part of a wider programme are yarrow and other **peripheral vasodilators,** buckwheat and **nervous restoratives.**

---

styptic, a remedy that stops bleeding and discharge; essentially a strong **astringent.**

---

sudorific, a remedy that produces profuse sweating, *see* **diaphoretic.**

---

sundew, Dewplant, *Drosera rotundifolia* L. Fam: Droseraceae.

A small herb with long-stalked round leaves covered on the upper surface with long red hairs with small glands on the tips; the white flowers are arranged in a unilateral raceme at the end of smooth, slender flowerstems up to 15cm high — they open out in the sunlight.

Habitat: in bogs and wet ground throughout Britain, Europe, northern Asia and North America.

Constituents: naphthaquinones (including plumbatin).

Actions: relaxing expectorant; antispasmodic; demulcent.

Applications: to asthmatic conditions and dry, tickly or nervous cough; to tracheitis and whooping cough and other respiratory conditions marked by viscid mucus; to gastric inflammation and ulceration.

Dosage: 0.5-2 grams of dried herb equivalent three times per day.

---

suppositories, small cones made of a suspension of medicine in a soft base readily dissolved at body temperature (cocoa butter is a traditional material), so as to provide a convenient method of applying medicines via the rectum.

---

sweet flag, Calamus, Sweet sedge, *Acorus calamus* L. Fam: Araceae.

The rhizome of a reed-like plant with linear leaves 60-100cm long; the flowering stem is simple and erect and flattened with a dense lateral yellow-green flower spike 5-8cm long; the odour of the rhizome is sweet and aromatic.

Habitat: water edges over temperate regions of the northern hemisphere.

Constituents: volatile oil (including asarone, eugenol, asamyl alcohol); a bitter principle (acorin); tannin; mucilage.

Actions: relaxing tonic to the upper digestive tract; carminative.

Applications: to nervous and acid dyspeptic conditions, including hyperacidity and peptic ulceration; intestinal colic and flatulence; anorexia and digestive incompetence.

Dosage: 0.5-2 grams of the dried rhizome equivalent three times per day.

Caution: it is unwise to exceed the stated dose of this remedy and the isolated oil should never be used.

Swertia chirata,   chiretta.

Symphytum officinale,   comfrey.

Symplocarpus foetidus,   skunk cabbage.

---

syrup,   solutions of sugar and water that are often used to preserve and act as a vehicle for herbal extracts; they are particularly suited to children and for disguising obnoxious tastes.

Syzygium cumini,   jambul.

T

---

tablets,   compressed preparations of medicaments with binding agents, and other substances designed to aid in digesting and assimilating the contents; flavourings and colourings are often added in the commercial processes used, although this is far less likely with herbal tablets.

Tanacetum parthenium,   feverfew.

Tanacetum vulgare,   tansy.

---

tannins,   phenolic plant constituents found most prominently in tissues outside active plant metabolism (e.g., old and dying leaves outer cork.

heartwood and galls) possibly as waste products, but with pest repellent activity as well; they have been used through the ages to tan animal hides to make leather, as their effect when encountering protein is to curdle it (in much the same way as boiling curdles egg-white); their effect on the body is **astringent**.

---

tansy, *Tanacetum vulgare* L. *Chrysanthemum vulgare* (L) Bernh. Fam: Compositae.

A stout erect perennial up to 1 metre high with creeping rootstock; the large pinnate leaves are deeply divided into toothed segments; numerous golden-yellow flowerheads occur in a large terminal corymb; the odour is strongly camphoraceous and the taste is bitter.

Habitat: waysides, field borders and waste ground throughout Britain, Europe, Asia and North America.

Constituents: volatile oil (including thujone), sesquiterpene lactones (including santonin), miscellaneous terpenoids (including artemisia ketone and the pyrethrins), bitter glycosides, flavonoids, tannins and resin.

Actions: vermifuge and insecticidal; digestive stimulant; uterine stimulant; anti-spasmodic.

Applications: to nematode infestations in the gut; locally for scabies and for pruritus ani when asociated with gut infestations; gastro-enteric infections in general.

Dosage: 0.5-2 grams of dried herb equivalent three times per day.

Caution: tansy is potentially toxic and its use is not recommended for the untrained; it must never be used in pregnancy.

Taraxacum officinale et spp,   dandelion.

Teucrium chamaedrys,   germander, wall.

Teucrium scorodonia,   wood sage.

---

throat problems,   sore throats, whether pharyngitis, **tonsillitis,** or another specific problem, may be treated both locally, by gargles, and systemically. Remedies for gargles such as myrrh, balm of Gilead, marigold, thyme and sage (all best in tincture form), **astringent** remedies such as blackberry and raspberry leaves, catechu, avens, bistort, oak bark, cranesbill, rhatany, rose hips, tormentil, white pond lily, and soothing **demulcent** remedies such as marshmallow, ribwort, comfrey and licorice. Many of these remedies are likely to be quickly effective in both soothing and clearing the problem but parallel systemic treatment will often be useful for complete correction: **anti-infective** remedies such as wild indigo and echinacea and the **lymphatic** and **alterative** remedies will be among the first in mind, but the association of sore throats with a large number of wider problems must be considered. On the other hand the potential of infected throats to lead to far-reaching complications almost anywhere in the body increases the need for complete and speedy treatment.

thrombosis, the formation of clots in the bloodstream, so that they block the vessel, or as emboli, travel around the circulation to lodge somewhere else. Most common forms are cerebral thrombosis **(stroke)**, coronary thrombosis, a cause of heart attacks, pulmonary thrombosis or embolism, and thrombophlebitis (where the clot occurs in a vein, most often in the leg). Herbal treatment is usually considered after the event, as a contribution to measures to prevent re-occurrence. The problem is that anticoagulant drugs are almost always already being taken, and it is irresponsible to distort their 'knife-edge' action with other remedies. It is however possible to follow the basic regime as for **arteriosclerosis,** and for qualified practitioners only, to consider the use of limeflowers, hawthorn and other **peripheral vasodilators.** Garlic is almost always tolerated.

thrush, infection with a yeast, *Candida albicans*, occurring most frequently in the mouth, vagina (*see* **vaginal problems**), and increasingly in the large bowel. Often considered as a sign of lowered vitality, and restorative remedies should be a priority in treatment, combined with an effectively **convalescent** regime. Mouth infections can be treated with mouth washes of marigold, myrrh and echinacea, vaginal problems with douches and hormonal correction where necessary; bowel infections, accounting for many cases of food intolerances, flatulence, colic and disturbed bowel function, are more difficult to treat directly, but attention to digestive and liver function with **bitter** and other appropriate remedies, fasting followed by fresh garlic administration, and strong **astringent** remedies may be tried as part of a co-ordinated programme.

Thuja occidentalis, arbor-vitae.

thyme, common, *Thymus vulgaris* L. Fam: Labiatae.

A perennial low aromatic shrub with much-branched woody stems forming dense tufts from which arise tiny paired opposite leaves on short stalks, each with two minute leaflets at the base; the flowers are arranged in whorls in the axils of the upper leaves, of a typical labiate appearance, pink to lilac in colour. The odour is characteristic.

Habitat: indigenous to Mediterranean regions and southern Europe, but widely grown throughout the world, where it prospers almost anywhere in temperate climes.

Constituents: volatile oil (including thymol, borneol, pinene, linalool, carvacrol); bitter principle; saponins; flavonoids; tannins.

Actions: a relaxing antiseptic expectorant; antispasmodic; carminative and digestive tonic; locally antiseptic and astringent.

Applications: for relaxing and making fluid respiratory conditions marked by tension, dryness and irritability, including asthmatic symptoms; for children's respiratory conditions, enuresis and diarrhoea; for chronic gastric inflammations; an excellent mouthwash for gum disease; for throat infections as a gargle.

Dosage: 1-4 grams dried herb equivalent three times per day.

---

thyme, wild, Serpyllum, Wild thyme, *Thymus serpyllum* L. Fam: Labiatae.

A perennial low aromatic shrub resembling the common thyme but with a creeping rooting stem sending up erect shoots, with broader leaves with prominent veins on the undersurface, and with crowded flowerheads; the odour is slightly more lemon-like.

Habitat: native to Britain, Europe and northern and central Asia, on banks and dry hilly pastures.

Constituents: volatile oil (including cymol, carvacrol, thymol, pinene); bitter (serpyllin); tannin; flavonoids.

Actions: a stimulating expectorant with antispasmodic properties; antiseptic; diuretic.

Applications: for bronchial infections to soothe the cough and aid in the more efficient expulsion of the congested phlegm; for colic and flatulence; for some cases of painful menstruation; as a gargle and mouthwash for throat and mouth infection and inflammation.

Dosage: 0.5-4 grams of dried herb equivalent three times per day.

Thymus serpyllum, thyme, wild.

Thymus vulgaris, thyme, common.

---

thyroid disease, manifested by alterations in metabolic rate, nervous tone, appetite and weight gain, enlargement of the thyroid gland in the neck ('goitre'), and/or bulging staring eyes; the exact diagnosis and determination of thyroid disease must depend on modern clinical tests. The herbal approach is as always to treat the whole person and thus all possible background factors: as far as the thyroid itself is concerned kelp is generally considered as an almost universal tonic.

Tilia europaea, limeflowers.

---

tincture, a preparation made by steeping plant material in a mixture of alcohol and water. As this is done at room temperature a far longer steeping time is necessary than with a hot infusion (*see* **infusion**), and up to two weeks will be required. The advantages however are that shelf life is very long (at least a year and often longer), that much better extraction of some constituents (notably alkaloids, volatile oils and resins) is possible in the alcohol fraction, and that it is easier to produce a concentrated extract than with aqueous preparations. The herb is usually added to the liquid in the proportion of one part (metric weight) to five parts (metric volume), although 1:10 may also be used. The proportion of alcohol in the liquid varies from 25-90 per cent and depends on what constituents in the plant are deemed most important to extract: for most common herbs 25 per cent alcohol is quite satisfactory. (*See also* **extract.**)

---

tinnitus, or ringing in the ears, caused either by problems in the inner ear and/or balance organs (*see* **vertigo**), or by catarrh or inflammation in the middle ear chamber (*see* **ear problems**). The latter is much more likely to be treatable than the former.

---

tonic, a remedy that restores tone to the system; seen as essentially nourishing, supportive and restorative, thus not as dramatic in effect as the simple **stimulant,** but producing a much more sure, lasting benefit. In practice tonics have often combined **bitter** stimulation of digestion, assimilation and liver function, **alterative** and **eliminative** remedies, **circulatory stimulants,** with remedies that genuinely appear to have nourishing or supportive action on specific areas. **Nervous restoratives** are an important group of such remedies, and dandelion root, kelp, lucerne, vervain, damiana, poplar, slippery elm, betony, agrimony, helonias root and kola may all find particular application in specific conditions. It is important to note, however, that a tonic quality is an essential ingredient of the *majority* of herbal remedies most frequently used; in other words, it is a central feature of herbal treatment that the vital reserves are constantly repleted as far as possible: that no real progress to health can occur unless basic 'battery power' is maintained or replenished; most plants used in medicine have background qualities that effectively support their primary action along the lines mentioned above, e.g., chamomile not only relaxes and calms, but is a digestive stimulant and peripheral vasodilator.

---

tonsillitis, infection of the tonsils, lymphatic glands in the throat; most common in children. Removal of these important structures should only be a measure of last resort, and persistent problems at least should be viewed as a sign of excessive airborne or diet-linked challenges to the body's defence systems. In other words the causes of chronic tonsillitis should be sought in much wider areas than purely the throat. Local treatment will be similar to other throat infections (*see* **throat problems**), but expert advice will be necessary to eliminate the possibility of **quinsy** or **diphtheria**.

---

tormentil, Bloodroot, Septfoil, *Potentilla erecta* (L) Rausch., *P. tormentilla* L. Fam: Rosaceae.

The rootstock of a small creeping herb, hugging the ground underneath other ground cover, producing at intervals erect stems with stalked lower, and sessile upper leaves of the classic 'cinquefoil' shape (five-lobed: three main leaflets and two stipules); the flowers are in loose terminal tymes on long slender pedicels, with four petals, bright yellow; the roots are brown, internally reddish, with many scars, pits and elevations, and attachments to numerous filamentous rootlets.

Habitat: throughout Britain, Europe, western Asia and north Africa in pastures, open woods, and moorlands, particularly in light, acid soils.

Constituents: tannin (up to 20 per cent), red pigment, bitter glycoside, resin and gums.

Actions: one of the surest and safest astringent remedies in common use, particularly applicable to the gut wall.

Applications: to enteric irritation and inflammation, particularly that resulting in diarrhoea; to inflammation and ulceration of the colon (as symptomatic relief); to gastritis and peptic ulceration (to prevent exacerbation by food); as a mouthwash for pharyngeal affections and aphthous ulcers; locally as a lotion for haemorrhoids, as a vaginal douche and for cuts and discharging sores.

Dosage: 1-4 grams of dried root equivalent three times per day before meals.

---

traditional medicine, a term used to denote those forms of medicine practised in communities unaffected by modern technological developments; used particularly by the World Health Organization (WHO) in its programme designed to improve health in the Third World. In practice consists of a number of techniques, with a large shamanistic element, but the use of medicinal plants is by far the most prominent feature: this acts as a vast resource of human experience for those interested in researching the application of plant remedies in modern times (*see* **ethnopharmacology**).

---

travel sickness, nausea and vomiting brought on by the effect of motion on the balance organs in the middle ear; especially likely at menstruation, or with sinusitis, migraine or hypertension sufferers. Can be kept to a minimum by eating only simple foods and drinks, avoiding reading, keeping the windows open and keeping an eye on the horizon. Fresh ginger root is an ideal preventative chewed before and during travel in small pieces. Commercial travel pills are derived from a constituent of the henbane and deadly nightshade family — these plants are dangerous and should not be taken.

Trifolium pratense, red clover.

Trigonella foenum-graecum, fenugreek.

Trillium erectum, beth root.

Triticum repens, couch grass.

Turnera diffusa, damiana.

Tussilago farfara, coltsfoot.

U

ulcer, mouth, (aphthous ulcer), painful blisters and ulcers on the lining of the mouth, gums and tongue; small and bordered with red. Often found in association with debility, tendency to catch colds or other infections, digestive upsets, or friction from a jagged tooth. Mouthwashes with **astringent** herbs and antiseptic herbal tinctures such as myrrh, marigold, thyme, coupled with frequent teeth-cleaning will keep the local area clear; the condition will often improve on its own, but if it is linked with underlying debilities these will have to be treated properly.

ulcer, peptic, slow-healing erosion in the wall of stomach or duodenum ('gastric' or 'duodenal' respectively). Causes little known: those in the stomach associated with poor nutrition, smoking and excess alcohol intake, duodenal notably with 'executive stress', and both with **hyperacidity**; however there are always other complex factors as well. Should be checked as a possibility with *any* chronic pain associated with or following food. Treatment involves rest, use of **relaxant** remedies, and other measures to control hyperacidity; gastric ulcers may be improved by the use of healing agents such as licorice, marshmallow root, meadowsweet, comfrey and slippery elm. Duodenal ulcers are much harder to reach directly, but licorice is potentially useful. Treatment of some of the deeper causative factors will need professional herbal attention.

ulcer, varicose, erosion of varying size on the lower part of the leg, often associated with varicose veins, but always with chronically poor return of circulation from the area. Stagnation of the accumulated blood leads to progressive breakdown of the tissues and skin: the ulcer represents the actual breaking point. Typically very slow to heal and easy to spread. Treatment must emphasize the flushing through of the area: keep leg muscles moving with foot and toe exercises, keep feet up as much as possible, avoid standing around. Internally **circulatory stimulants** and **vascular remedies** are indicated, as well as marigold and comfrey; externally the priority is expert dressing, and professional nursing care is usually essential. **Astringent** and healing herbs may be applied as sterile **mucilaginous preparations** or dry powders.

Ulmus fulva, slippery elm.

---

unicorn root, false, *see* **helonias root.**

---

urethritis, *see* **urinary infections.**

Urginea maritima, squill.

---

urinary antiseptic, a remedy that whilst being excreted through the urinary system acts locally to disinfect the tubules. Herbal remedies of this type have a most beneficial and long-lasting application to **urinary infections** such as cystitis, especially when used for a few weeks after the main symptoms have gone: not only do they inhibit infective colonization of the tubules, but they appear to promote genuine healing of the mucosa so as to reduce the chances of re-infection, which is the principal problem with drug treatment. Most urinary antiseptics are safe, but a few can irritate the kidney and so all should be applied only after advice from a qualified herbal practitioner. The list includes uva-ursi, buchu, juniper, kava-kava, boldo, saw palmetto, celery seed, parsley seed, shepherd's purse, golden rod, heather flowers and pipsissewa.

---

urinary infections, specific infection, with inflammation, of the inner lining of the urinary system; if primarily affecting the bladder, known as cystitis, if the urinary outlet, urethritis; it may also move up to involve the tubules draining from the kidneys, ureteritis, or even the kidney itself, pyelitis or **phelonephritis**. Most likely to affect women, but not uncommon in men. The symptoms vary, especially with the site of infection, but usually include frequency, with irritation or scalding pain on passing water, possibly blood, pus or mucus passed, and, especially with urethritis, local pain and itching on penis or vulva. Fever may be present. The higher the site of the infection, the more likely that the pain will move up from the groin area round the side to the mid-back (the loins), that there will be fever (often severe), and that the urine will be scanty. Urinary infections may be contracted from external contamination (especially in women), or may even be **venereal** in origin, or may arise from any factor that reduces flow through the system, e.g., **prostatic disease, urinary stones,** or growths. Similarly such infection will be exacerbated by any factor slowing the flow of urine, and the first priority in treatment is to increase the dilution and flow: large quantities of fluid should be drunk, there should be a high intake of fruit and fruit juice, and herbal **diuretics** are indicated. On the whole alcohol, however, is more irritating than helpful. Other associated conditions must be treated as encountered, then a choice from the specific **urinary antiseptics** may be made, these taken for some weeks after the symptoms have gone to prevent reoccurrence. In women cystitis is often concurrent with, and occasionally confused with, **vaginal infections:** these must be treated as well.

Caution: if there is any possibility that the kidneys have been affected then the condition must be referred to a qualified practitioner. If there is any possibility that the infection is venereal in origin, then it must by U.K. law be referred to a doctor.

---

urinary stones,   the deposition in the urine of relatively insoluble excretory materials, most often salts of calcium. These crystallize when their concentration in the urine exceeds their solubility, either because too much is being excreted, or because the urine has become too concentrated itself, or because of changes in acidity, alkalinity or other chemical composition of the urine. In practice, stones will only form where the lining of the urinary mucosa is damaged, and the possibility of a parallel **urinary infection** should be considered. Symptoms vary from a sensation of mild 'grittiness' on passing urine, through to signs of blood (perhaps making the urine appear 'smoky'), to severe pain in any area from loin to groin. Small stones or 'gravel' may easily be passed, but larger deposits may require surgical removal. Herbal treatment concentrates on keeping the urine dilute (*see also* **urinary infections**), with **diuretics** (some of which have particular reputations for helping with this condition), and dealing with background factors as far as possible. Depending on the type of stone dietary adjustment is often possible.

Urtica dioica et spp,   nettle.

---

uterine remedies, those remedies most likely to be used for gynaecological and occasionally obstetric problems; the term is preferred to **emmenogogues,** but does not include **hormonal remedies,** which are usually an intrinsic part of gynaecological treatment (*see* **women's remedies**). Many stimulate the uterus and are contra-indicated in pregnancy, but others are more tonifying and even relaxing; it is necessary to choose from the following list those most appropriate to the particular condition: beth root, black haw, blue cohosh, celery, chamomile, cinchona, cotton root, feverfew, lady's mantle, life root, motherwort, mugwort, parsley, pasque flower, pennyroyal, raspberry, rue, southernwood, squaw vine, white deadnettle and yarrow.

---

uva-ursi, Bearberry, Mountain cranberry, Sandberry, *Arctostaphylos uva-ursi* Spreng. Fam: Ericaceae.

The leaves of a small evergreen creeping shrub; the leaves are shiny oblong, with entire margins up to 2.5cm long; the flowers are in drooping terminal racemes, small, pink-to-white, bell-shaped, and in groups of four to six, giving way to globular bright red berries.

Habitat: on dry rocky hills over the northern regions of the northern hemisphere, often very extensive ground cover.

Constituents: glycosides (including arbutin, methyl-arbutin and ericolin); resin (ursone); flavonoids; tannins.

Actions: owing to conversion of arbutin to the antiseptic hydroquinone in the urinary tubules, a potent and selective urinary antiseptic particularly in highly acidic urine; astringent effect on the lower digestive tract.

Applications: to infections of the urinary tract especially associated with acidic urine, though probably to be avoided if the kidney itself is affected.

Dosage: 1-4 grams of dried leaves equivalent three times per day.

V

---

vaccination, the herbalist shares with other practitioners of natural medicine some degree of doubt about the conventional practice of vaccination: this varies from outright rejection of the idea of injecting toxic material into the system to a more pragmatic realization that the practice has validity in certain areas. This more balanced view still asserts strongly that the healthy body has enormous defence resources at its disposal, and that too ready a reliance on vaccination reduces the responsibility we have to maintain health positively; further, vaccination is not always effective; however, there are some people and communities where the chance of furthering positive health is low and there vaccinations have an established effect. For each disease vaccinated against it is possible to develop a positive strategy, e.g., *see* **whooping cough** *and* **poliomyelitis,** using herbs at various stages to reduce the chance of contracting the full diseases. For the treatment of vaccination side-effects the herb arbor-vitae is specifically recommended, though other **alteratives** are applicable.

---

vaginal problems,   the vagina normally keeps infection at bay by playing host to beneficial bacteria (Döderlein's bacilli), providing them with glucose which they convert to lactic acid and so acidify the vaginal interior, to the discomfiture of other influences. Loss of this protection is due to poor oestrogen influence on the cells of the vaginal wall, thus may follow use of the Pill or may be a sign of other hormonal disruption. Any such factor must be treated first, and helonias root may be indicated for internal treatment. After internal factors have been attended to, external herbal treatment can then be applied, infusions or decoctions of herbs in douche form. Prime remedies are periwinkle, beth root, marigold, arbor-vitae, myrrh, white pond lily, witch hazel and most astringent remedies. In former times the discharges accompanying vaginal infections such as Candida (or thrush), were known as 'leucorrhoea' or 'whites' and were seen as catarrhal or cleansing symptoms. Eliminative or **alterative** remedies would thus be prescribed, and the possibility of congestive conditions in the lower abdomen investigated. It is also wise to consider the possibility of **urinary infection** and treat that concurrently. A dry, irritating vaginitis occasionally occurs after **menopause;** it may be treated locally with demulcent and healing herbs. *See also* **cervical problems.**

---

valerian,   All-heal, *Valeriana officinalis* L. Fam: Valerianaceae.
The roots of a perennial herb up to 1.5 metres in height, with erect, fluted stems. Pinnate leaves with large lanceolate segments; the rootstock is short giving off a tuft of long creeping runners; the stems terminate in broad corymbs of numerous flowers, white tinged with pink, funnel-shaped with five unequal lobes. The fresh runners are odourless but, on drying, develop the characteristic pungent smell. The plant is not to be confused with the

common red 'American' valerian.

Habitat: in moist situations, on the banks of streams or ditches over the whole of Europe up to the Arctic circle; it is naturalized in the eastern U.S.A.

Constituents: volatile oil (including valerianic acid, borneol, pinene, camphene, and assorted sesquiterpenes); volatile alkaloids (chatinine, valerianine, skythantine); iridoids (the sedative valepotriates, though possibly only in the fresh plant); resins and gums.

Actions: tranquillizer, antispasmodic, expectorant, diuretic, warming.

Applications: to anxiety states, insomnia, all conditions of nervous tension, calming without being notably sedative and practically non-addictive; its lack of depressing properties supported by the fact that traditionally it was its healing, warming, expectorant and diuretic actions that were commended, and it was used as a veritable heal-all (hence a common name); locally applied it is effective for cramps and other muscle tensions.

Dosage: 1-4 grams of the fresh or dried root equivalent three times a day.

Valeriana officinalis, valerian.

---

varicose veins, swollen and stretched veins in the legs (or rectum: *see* **haemorrhoids**) caused by a combination of poor venous return to the heart, extra abdominal pressure from above (obesity, constipation, pregnancy, shallow breathing), and congenitally weakened vein walls. Improved exercise will help the leg muscles pump the veins clear of congestion (especially if combined with raising the legs whenever possible); treatment should concentrate on relieving other factors; herbal remedies that will help on internal treatment include horse chestnut, golden seal, limeflowers and stone root; externally marigold, stone root or horse chestnut may be massaged into the tissues affected.

---

vascular remedies, herbs that appear to act to improve the health of the blood vessels, in for example capillary fragility, petechiae and, more contentiously, in **arteriosclerosis, varicose veins, migraine** and other vascular diseases. Most include quantities of **flavonoid glycosides**. Notable examples are buckwheat, rue, (horse) chestnut and limeflowers.

---

venereal disease, any condition transmitted by or resulting from sexual contact. It is to be suspected in *any* urinary, vaginal or cervical condition, particularly associated with external sores in the genital area. As well as the main groups of gonorrhoea and syphilis, a wide group of conditions are known to be sexually-transmitted in some cases, including trichomoniasis, vaginal fungal infections, non-specific urethritis, and Reiter's disease. It is an offence in the U.K. for anyone other than a registered medical practitioner to treat or prescribe remedies for any venereal disease.

Verbascum thapsus, mullein.

Verbena officinalis, vervain.

---

vermifuge, *see* **anthelmintic.**

Veronica virginica, black root.

Veronicastrum virginicum, black root.

---

vertigo, or dizziness, is a disturbance in the balance mechanism of the middle ear, most often brought on by loss of blood supply to the area; thus associated with loss of fluid and electrolytes by excessive sweating in unaccustomed hot weather (when typically seen on sudden rising), or more chronically, with **arteriosclerosis** and **high blood-pressure;** may also follow middle **ear problems,** Meniere's disease, **migraine** or **epilepsy.** A symptom rather than a disease, but may be helped a little by betony and fresh ginger if persistent.

---

vervain, Verbena, *Verbena officinalis* L. Fam: Verbenaceae.

A slender, erect perennial 30-90cm high with a central, almost hairless, stem and many long thin branches; the lower leaves are deeply divided and stalked, the upper ones slender and sessile and toothed; tiny white flowers appear in long slender spikes.

Habitat: waysides and wasteplaces in central and southern Europe, Asia and southern Britain, and as an escape elsewhere in the world.

Constituents: glycosides (including verbenin, verbenalin); bitter principle; volatile oil; tannin; alkaloid.

Actions: relaxant; tonic; galactogogue; diaphoretic.

Applications: as a calming restorative for debilitated conditions and particularly nervous exhaustion; as an antispasmodic in asthmatic, migrainous and other symptoms of visceral tension; as a component of a fever-management regime; to promote increased milk production; as a component of hepatic prescriptions; as an excellent mouthwash for dental and gum diseases.

Dosage: 1-4 grams of dried herb equivalent three times per day.

---

vesicants, remedies that provoke blister formation on application to the skin; essentially very strong **rubefacients** that were used to provide drastically increased blood supply to an inflamed area, with the extra effect of producing a fluid discharge, initially into a blister, but when this is punctured (as is usual), producing a free flow for some considerable time. Traditionally this fluid was assumed to contain toxic matter from the inflamed site (an arthritic joint in most cases), and it is a matter of record that the technique was able to produce quite dramatic alleviation of the condition (e.g., freedom from even severe symptoms of arthritis for a considerable time). Blistering, however, is a skilled technique, not now widely performed in modern practice, and it is to be emphasized that it is potentially dangerous in unskilled hands. Vesicant remedies are inherently irritant in nature and include croton oil, turpentine, cowhage and formic acid.

Viburnum opulus, cramp bark.

Viburnum prunifolium, black haw.

Vinca major, periwinkle, greater.

Viola odorata, violet, sweet.

Viola tricolor, heartsease.

---

violet, sweet, English violet, Garden violet, Blue violet, *Viola odorata* L. Fam: Violaceae.

A perennial herb with a thick, short rhizome, knotted and branched with the remains of old leafstalks and stipules, producing a rosette of stalked, broadly-cordate leaves with crenate margins; the long-stemmed violet-coloured or white flowers are five-petalled with a short spur on the lower petal; there is a delicate scent.

Habitat: on banks and hedges, field borders and woods, patchily distributed around Britain, Europe, Asia, and in the region of cultivated gardens elsewhere in the world: it is very unobtrusive and easy to miss among other plants.

Constituents: saponins, methyl salicylate, alkaloid (odoratine or violine), essential oil, flavonoids.

Actions: anti-inflammatory, stimulating **expectorant**; diuretic; antineoplastic.

Applications: to congestive pulmonary conditions; as a useful background influence in the treatment of carcinoma, especially affecting the breast, lungs and alimentary canal; as a mouthwash for infections of the mouth and throat.

Dosage: 1-6 grams of dried herb equivalent three times a day.

Viscum album, mistletoe.

Vitex agnus-castus, agnus-castus.

---

volatile oils, mixtures of hydrocarbons, prominently terpenes, with a strong odour, less soluble in water than fat and alcohol, obviously produced by many herbal remedies; they have many pharmacological actions so that it pays to take steps in preparing herbal preparations not to lose too much volatile oil in the atmosphere; many stimulate peripheral circulation (*see* **peripheral vasodilators** *and* **circulatory stimulants**), others taste **bitter,** several are **antiseptic,** many are **carminative, antispasmodic** and **relaxant,** through both local effects on the sensory nerves of the gut and systemic action. It is relatively easy to judge the extent of volatile oil content by the smell of the sample. Notable isolated volatile oils are menthol (from the mint family), camphor (as in feverfew, tansy and some of the wormwood family), thymol (a strongly antiseptic constituent of thyme and other labiate plants), thujone (from sage), borneol, pinene and cineol.

---

vomiting,   may arise directly from the stomach, or from stimulation of the vomiting centre in the brain. Many causes the same as for **nausea,** also glaucoma, cerebral infection or tumour, Ménière's disease, skull injuries and several general diseases; nervous vomiting may be encountered, especially in children ('cyclic vomiting') and in **bulimia nervosa.** Treatment as for nausea, with the use of **relaxants** such as chamomile, lemon balm and particularly horehound (black).

---

vulnerary,   a remedy used for healing wounds; *see* **astringent** and **healing remedies.**

W

---

warts,   or verrucae, are virally-induced overgrowths of the epidermis of the skin; occur almost anywhere and usually without explanation, although they are mildly contagious by contact (genital warts can be spread by venereal contact for example). They are inherently non-serious but can be a nuisance and disfiguring. It is always worth checking for internal causes and factors (as with **eczema** for example): externally they are sometimes removed with direct contact by the milky sap of the fresh dandelion root, the orange sap of the celandine, or tincture of arbor-vitae, in all cases such administration to be repeated frequently for days or even weeks.

---

white deadnettle,   Blind nettle, Archangel, *Lamium album* L. Fam: Labiatae.

The flowering tops of this nettle-like plant, but with labiate-like, square hollow stems and white labiate flowers in close axillary whorls of six to ten or more.

Habitat: on banks and hedgerows in waste places throughout Britain, Europe and Asia, as well as eastern U.S.A.

Constituents: flavonoids, tannins, essential oil, mucilage, monoamines, choline.

Actions: astringent antispasmodic for the female reproductive system,

215

improving uterine bloodflow when defective, and appearing to encourage a co-ordinated uterine muscular activity; a prostatic remedy.

Applications: menstrual difficulties, especially menorrhagia, discharges and other symptoms of a congestive condition of the pelvis; for prostatic ailments under the same conditions; to spasmodic or congestive dysmenorrhoea.

Dosage: 1-4 grams of the dried herb equivalent three times per day.

---

white pond lily (American), Water nymph, Water cabbage, Cow cabbage, *Nymphaea odorata* Soland. Fam: Nymphaeaceae.

The rhizome of an aquatic perennial plant with large orbicular or oblong-orbicular entire leaves floating on the water surface and large white flowers opening in late morning every day for three days; the rhizome is obtained in pieces up to 5cm in diameter, greyish-brown to black externally, yellowish or greyish-white internally, starchy in texture with an interrupted sub-cortical ring; the taste is mucilaginous and slightly pungent.

Habitat: in ponds and slow streams in eastern North America.

Constituents: not well established

Actions: a demulcent and astringent; antiseptic.

Applications: to the management of diarrhoea and checking enteritis; locally as a douche for cervical discharge, as a gargle for throat infections, and as a poultice for boils.

Dosage: 1-2 grams of dried rhizome equivalent three times per day.

---

whitlow, *see* **abscess.**

---

whooping cough, an infection of the mucous membranes of the airways, producing a notably sticky tenuous mucus; the result is a distressing, convulsive cough, leading to breathlessness and the characteristic 'whoop'; most often affects children, and potentially dangerous before the age of three; a difficult infection to dislodge so aim is to reduce the symptoms, especially the tendency to vomiting, and the duration of the illness. Mainly a job for professional practitioners who will use a careful blend of **expectorants,** stimulating or relaxing according to the situation. Thyme, licorice, elecampane, mullein flowers and occasionally lobelia may be used in this way. **Relaxant** remedies may always be applied for the convulsions and distress. Main priority is to keep the patient warm, but with good fresh air as much as possible. This condition must not be neglected. *Prevention* against whooping cough is best accomplished by preventing stuffy damp rooms and working positively to contain cold attacks.

---

wild cherry bark, Virginian prune, *Prunus serotina* Ehrh. Fam: Rosaceae.

The bark of a large tree (up to 30 metres) with alternate stiff oblong or ovate leaves with serrated margins and small white flowers growing in lateral racemes; the bark is rough and nearly black on older trunks, but that used is younger, smooth and glossy and reddish-brown, with white lenticels, with underlying greenish-brown cortex; the taste is astringent and bitter, recalling bitter almonds when wet.

Habitat: in woods through eastern, central and northern North America.

Constituents: cyanogenic glycosides, volatile oil, coumarins, benzoic acid, gallitannins, resin.

Actions: antitussive; mild sedative; digestive stimulant; astringent.

Applications: to irritable and painful cough when increasing expectoration is inappropriate; to the racking or exhausting cough of debility or convalescence.

Dosage: 0.5-2 grams of dried bark equivalent three times per day.

---

wild indigo, Horsefly weed, Yellow indigo, *Baptisia tinctoria* R.Br. Fam: Leguminosae.

The root of a perennial plant up to 1.3 metres in height, with erect, slender branches bearing alternate greyish-green trilobular leaves with three obovate leaflets and bright-yellow leguminous flowers in loose terminal racemes; the root is externally roughened, grooved and warty, with, internally, a yellowish-brown fibrous core easily separating from the thick bark; the taste is bitter and acrid.

Habitat: in dry soil of woods and clearings of central and eastern North America.

Constituents: alkaloids (including baptitoxin), purgative glycosides (including baptin), flavonoids (including baptisin), resin.

Actions: circulatory stimulant; anti-infective; alterative; cholagogue and laxative.

Applications: to infections and inflammations, especially affecting the tonsils, throat, lymphatic system, mouth; to boils and furunculosis; to containing fever associated with persistent or aggressive local infections; locally for ulcers, boils and any infection.

Dosage: 0.2-1 gram of dried root equivalent three times per day.

---

wild yam, Colic root, Rheumatism root, *Dioscorea villosa* L. Fam: Dioscoreaceae.

The rhizome of a twining perennial vine with ovate and cordate leaves, shiny above but finely hairy underneath, producing greenish-yellow flowers, the male in drooping panicles, the female in racemes; the rhizome is obtained as hard chips, yellowish, and paler inside; the taste is bitter with an acrid aftertaste.

Habitat: in thickets and hedges over eastern North America.

Constituents: steroidal saponins (including dioscine), phytosterols, alkaloids (including dioscorine), tannins and starch.

Actions: visceral relaxant and antispasmodic; mild peripheral vasodilator and diaphoretic; cholagogue; (possibly steroidal) anti-inflammatory.

Applications: to functional colitis, colonic spasm, and the symptoms of inflammatory colitis and dysentery; to colic; to diverticulitis; to cramps and intermittent claudication; to rheumatic inflammatory conditions.

Dosage: 1-4 grams of dried rhizome equivalent three times per day.

---

willow bark, European willow, *Salix alba* L. *et spp.* Fam: Salicaceae.

The bark of several species of willow, with slightly downy and finely serrulate leaves, and prominent catkins; the bark is obtained in thin channelled pieces, the outer surface smooth and glossy or wrinkled and rough, depending on its age, of a brown to greenish colour, the inner surface yellowish, reddish or brown and fibrous; the taste is astringent and bitter.

Habitat: throughout Britain and central and southern Europe, and widely cultivated elsewhere.

Constituents: salicylates (including salicin), condensed tannins.

Actions: anti-inflammatory and in other ways exhibiting salicylate activity; astringent and locally antiseptic; bitter digestive tonic.

Applications: to rheumatic inflammations and the inflammatory stages of auto-immune diseases; to check hyperpyrexia in fever management; to neuralgias and post-inflammatory pains in convalescence; in enteric and dysenteric disease.

Dosage: 0.5-3 grams of dried bark equivalent three times per day.

---

wind, *see* **flatulence.**

---

wintergreen, Teaberry, Checkerberry, *Gaultheria procumbens* L. Fam: Ericaceae.

The leaves and aerial stems of a low, evergreen shrub with subterranean creeping stems, growing to no more than 15cm high, with erect branches bearing alternate oval, serrated leathery leaves and solitary nodding white flowers near the top; the latter gives way to a scarlet berry-like capsule.

Habitat: underneath other, especially Ericaceous plants, in woodlands through north-eastern North America.

Constituents: salicylate glycoside (gaultherin).

Actions: anti-inflammatory; diuretic; carminative.

Applications: to rheumatoid arthritis, both locally and systemically.

Dosage: 0.5-1 gram of dried stem and leaves three times a day; oil of wintergreen is most often derived from a species of birch, and may be applied externally as a liniment.

---

witch hazel, *Hamamelis virginiana* L. Fam: Hamamelidaceae.

The bark or leaves of a small deciduous tree growing to a height of up to 5 metres with alternate elliptic, coarsely toothed leaves with prominent veins often finely hairy underneath; drooping axillary clusters of yellow flowers appear in the autumn when the leaves are falling and give way to a woody capsule ejecting two shiny black seeds the following year; the taste of both leaves and bark is astringent and bitter.

Habitat: in damp woodland throughout eastern and central North America.

Constituents: mixed tannins, a bitter principle, volatile oil.

Actions: astringent.

Applications: to enteric inflammation and infection; to contain bleeding and excessive mucous discharge from the alimentary canal; locally for haemorrhoids, bruises and wounds.

Dosage: 1-4 grams of dried bark or leaf equivalent three times per day.

Note: the distilled witch hazel widely sold is not as astringent as other preparations as no tannins are present.

---

women's remedies, herbal remedies have an enormous potential in gynaecological problems (perhaps not least since most traditional herbalists were women) and they offer many chances to treat both functional and organic disorders without hormone treatment or surgery; *see* **uterine remedies, hormonal remedies, menstrual disorders, menopause, pregnancy, labour, galactogogue, breast problems, fibroids** and other specific conditions.

---

wood sage, Garlic sage, *Teucrium scorodonia* L. Fam: Labiatae.

A perennial erect herb or shrub about 30cm high, slightly branched with narrow or ovate stalked leaves, roughly toothed, wrinkled and downy; pairs of pale-yellow flowers, each with a small bract on one side of the stem; there is a sage-like odour.

Habitat: in hedges and woods throughout Britain, Europe and northern Asia except in the extreme north.

Constituents: volatile oil, saponins, flavonoids, tannins.

Actions: gently warming diaphoretic; carminative; locally astringent and healing.

Applications: to feverish conditions and the common cold as part of a fever management strategy; to dyspeptic and flatulent conditions; as a local application for slow-healing wounds, boils and ulcers.

Dosage: 1-4 grams of the dried herb equivalent three times per day.

---

worms, intestinal, *see* **anthelmintics.**

---

wormwood, Absinthe, Green ginger, *Artemisia absinthium* L. Fam: Compositae.

An aromatic perennial plant with erect stems up to 1 metre tall, very tough, but dying back each autumn; the whole plant is greyish-white and covered with a fine down; the leaves are much dissected into fine lobes; the numerous flowerheads are arranged in dense racemose panicles, with heads drooping, nearly hemispherical, and yellow; the leaves taste extremely bitter with a characteristic odour.

Habitat: indigenous to maritime areas of Britain and Europe, but naturalized in many parts of the world on roadsides and waste places.

Constituents: volatile oil (including thujone, isovaleric acid); bitter sesquiterpene lactones of numerous types; terpenoids; flavonoids; triterpenoid; hydroxycoumarins; tannins, silica; resin.

Actions: one of the bitterest remedies in common use and thus a prime stimulant to digestion (see bitters); antiparasitic.

Applications: to digestive debility, anorexia and atonic gastritis; Enterobius and Ascaris infestations (but *see* **anthelmintics**).

Dosage: 1-2 grams dried herb equivalent three times per day before meals.

Y

yarrow, Milfoil, Nosebleed, Staunchgrass, *Achillea millefolium* L. Fam: Compositae.

The flowers of a perennial creeping herb with tough, erect, furrowed woody stems up to 0.5 metre high; the leaves are 5-12cm long, bi- and tri-pinnate, accounting for its Latin name meaning 'thousand-leaf'; the composite flowers are arranged in dense terminal corymbs, white to pink, each flower being about 4-6mm in diameter and with a characteristic odour.

Habitat: common in pastures, grassy banks, hedgerows and wasteplaces in dry sunny positions throughout much of the world.

Constituents: volatile oil (including cineol, azulene, eugenol, thujone, pinene, camphor); bitter constituents; cyanogenic glycosides; salicylates; aspargin; flavonoids; tannins; isovalerianic acid; resins.

Action: astringent, **peripheral vasodilator,** diaphoretic, digestive stimulant, antispasmodic, menstrual regulator.

Applications: widely regarded traditionally as a wound herb, especially in cases where these were poorly healing, and also used widely as a digestive remedy, improving appetite and settling digestion; it excels however in encouraging a redistribution of circulation to the periphery, especially during fever, and is one of the primary fever-management remedies — both the digestive action and relaxant effect are ideal accompaniments to the circulatory effect in feverish conditions; used also in controlling some cases of heavy menstrual bleeding and vaginal discharges.

Dosage: 1-4 grams of dried flowers equivalent three or more times a day.

yellow jasmine, *see* **gelsemium.**

Z

Zanthoxylum americanum, prickly ash.

Zea mays,   corn silk.

Zingiber officinale,   ginger.

USEFUL ADDRESSES

United States of America

American Herb Association
Box 353
Rescue, CA 95672

Mark Blumenthal
Herbalgram
P.O. Box 12602
Austin, TX 78711
(Tel: 512-385-6988)

Herb Research Foundation
Rob McCaleb, President
Box 2602
Longmont, CO 80501
(Tel: 303-449-2265)

L. D. Israelsen, Atty. at Law
P.O. Box 4000
Springville, UT 84663

United Kingdom
National Institute of Medical Herbalists
41 Hatherley Road
Winchester
Hampshire SO22 6RR

Australia
The Secretary
National Herbalists Association of Australia
49 Oakwood Street
Sutherland, NSW 2232